YOUR *pregnancy* BIBLE

SECOND
pregnancy

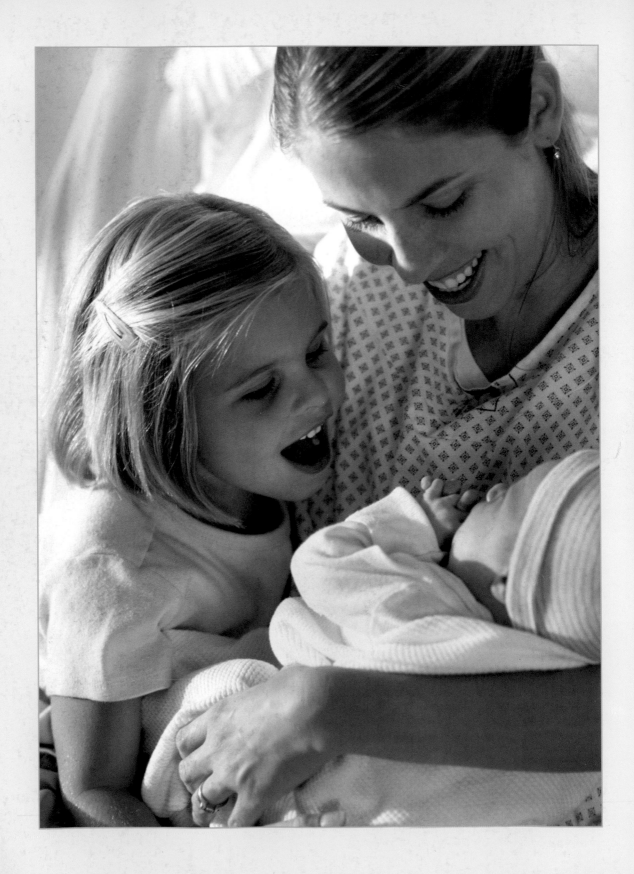

YOUR *pregnancy* BIBLE

SECOND

pregnancy

CONTRIBUTING EDITOR **Dr Penny Preston**

CARROLL & BROWN PUBLISHERS LIMITED

First published in 2010 in the United Kingdom by

Carroll & Brown Publishers Limited
20 Lonsdale Road
London NW6 6RD

Managing Art Editor Emily Cook
Photography Jules Selmes
Editorial Assistance Idroma Montgomery

Copyright © Carroll & Brown Limited 2010

A CIP catalogue record for this book is available
from the British Library.

ISBN 978 1 904 760 81 8

10 9 8 7 6 5 4 3 2 1

Reproduced by RALI, Spain
Printed and bound in China

CONTRIBUTORS

Penny Preston MB ChB, MRCGP, qualified as a doctor in 1989 and worked as a general practitioner for some years before becoming a health writer. She has contributed to numerous titles covering all areas of health and medicine, while having a special interest in pregnancy and child health.

Keith Eddleman, MD is a professor in the Department of Obstetrics, Gynaecology and Reproductive Sciences at the Mount Sinai School of Medicine in New York City. He is also the Director of Obstetrics at The Mount Sinai Hospital on Manhattan's Upper East Side. He is board-certified in OB/GYN, maternal-fetal medicine and clinical genetics. He was consulting editor for *The Pregnancy Bible* and was co-author of *Pregnancy for Dummie*s. In addition to practising medicine, he teaches medical students, residents and fellows. Keith also was involved with the acclaimed *Pregnancy for Dummies* series on the Discovery Health channel.

Joanne Stone, MD is a professor in the Department of Obstetrics, Gynaecology and Reproductive Sciences at the Mount Sinai School of Medicine in New York City as well as the Division Director and Fellowship Director of Maternal-Fetal Medicine. She was consulting editor of *The Pregnancy Bible* and co-author of *Pregnancy for Dummies* and was also featured in the *Pregnancy for Dummies* Discovery Health series.

r. Richard Woolfson, PhD, FBPS is a child sychologist and an honorary lecturer at the niversity of Strathcylde. He works with children and eir families. He has written books on child and mily psychology, and contributed both to *Your regnancy Bible* and *Your Babycare Bible*. He writes a eekly column in *The Herald* on parenting problems nd family issues, appears regularly on radio and television and runs workshops on child development.

Contents

Introduction

Stretch marks, sore nipples and swollen feet followed by nappy changes, sleepless nights and potty training – so you are thinking about doing this all over again? Really?

Are you sure you are ready again for the complete and utter joy of holding a newborn baby next to your body, with that wonderful baby smell unique to newborns, and feeling the immediate love for another human being and the unconditional love you get in return. Of course you are. There are few things in this world as incredibly special as having a baby. However, this time around, you have even more to think about: how a new baby will impact on your firstborn, how it will affect your work and marriage and how things might be different medically from your first pregnancy.

The original *Your Pregnancy Bible* was published in 2003 and has helped many expectant parents navigate their first pregnancy. The tremendous positive feedback received from readers, patients and even other doctors and midwives prompted an additional book addressing the specific need for information regarding a second pregnancy. There are many issues that uniquely pertain to a second or further pregnancy, which are not covered in sufficient depth in books geared to first pregnancies

---

Being pregnant

1st baby You begin wearing maternity clothes as soon as your pregnancy is confirmed.

2nd baby You wear your regular clothes for as long as possible.

3rd baby Your maternity clothes ARE your regular clothes.

Preparing for the birth

1st baby You practise your breathing religiously.

2nd baby You don't bother because you remember that last time, breathing didn't do a thing.

3rd baby You ask for an epidural in your eighth month.

The layette

1st baby You pre-wash newborn's clothes, colour-coordinate them, and fold them neatly in the baby's little bureau.

2nd baby You check to make sure that the clothes are clean and discard only the ones with the darkest stains.

3rd baby Boys can wear pink, can't they?

Worries

1st baby At the first sign of distress – a whimper or frown – you pick up your baby.

2nd baby When your baby's wails threaten to wake your firstborn, you pick your baby up.

3rd baby You teach your three-year-old how to rewind the mechanical swing.

– most obviously, how already having a child may impact on the experience!

There are physical changes, which are more dramatic in a second pregnancy including the greater fatigue some women feel since they not only are pregnant but have to keep up their energy to care for the child at home, and emotional worries such as how the birth of a second child may affect the feelings and behaviour of the first.

Many lifestyle issues may need to be considered, like the ideal timing to become pregnant, how to juggle caring for two (or more) and the financial implications. There are also some important medical considerations. If, for example, you had a caesarean birth the first time, should you try for a vaginal delivery and how a second labour might differ from the first.

Second Pregnancy also contains comprehensive information on exercise and diet, getting your home ready for a new child and strategies for using your time most efficiently. More than anything, it will serve as a guidebook, resource and companion for any questions, issues and concerns you may have the second time around! We hope this will give you encouragement, guidance and good advice and keep you on a positive and productive track towards your expanding family.

Finally, just to reassure you that second pregnancies and their resulting offspring are generally easier to manage, we'd like to leave you with a few observations from *pregnancytoday.com* about the likely outcome.

Activities

1st baby You take your infant to baby gymnastics, baby swing, baby zoo, baby movies and baby story hour.

2nd baby You take your infant to baby gymnastics.

3rd baby You take your infant to the supermarket and the dry cleaners.

Going out

1st baby The first time you leave your baby with a sitter, you call home five times.

2nd baby Just before you walk out the door, you remember to leave a number where you can be reached.

3rd baby You leave instructions for the sitter to call only if she sees blood.

At home

1st baby You spend a good bit of every day just gazing at the baby.

2nd baby You spend a bit of everyday watching to be sure your older child isn't squeezing, poking, or hitting the baby.

3rd baby You spend a little bit of every day hiding from your children.

Swallowing coins

1st child When first child swallows a coin, you rush the child to the hospital and demand x-rays.

2nd child When second child swallows a coin, you carefully watch for the coin to pass.

3rd child When your third child swallows a coin you deduct it from his pocket money!

1

ACHIEVING A SECOND PREGNANCY

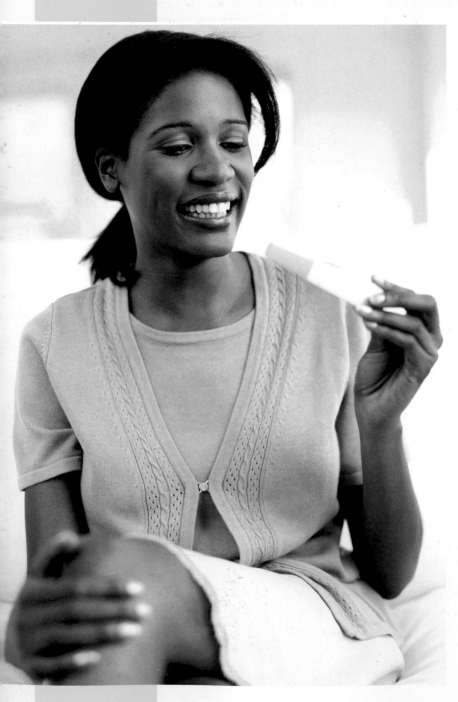

If you are reading this book it is because you have begun to embark on the exciting path of having a second (or third) child. Whereas the first time around there was only you and your partner's situation to consider, now there's another person whose entire future life will be affected by the decision you make. There will be many factors to consider and possibly treatment to undergo if conception doesn't happen as you'd wish.

Making the decision

Most people think hard when planning for another child. They have to take many factors – emotional, financial and practical – into consideration. On the other hand, sometimes the decision is taken out of one's hands – and that brings its own consequences.

Emotional considerations

You may wonder if you have had enough time alone with your first born, before embarking on another pregnancy. There is no absolute right or wrong answer to this question. Having a second child will definitely affect the time you have with your first child, but bear in mind the positives can outweigh any perceivable negatives. Realise that there will be ways to divide yourself so that you will be able to still spend some alone time with your first child (and later, with your second); for example, take advantage of family and friends who are willing to babysit. Also, be prepared that, depending on your child's age and personality, bringing home a new baby will have an effect on him. There's a reason why they call it "sibling rivalry", and it often stays around for a long time (see page 13). However, the bonds that your children make can be special and enduring and learning to deal with siblings can be an important and valuable lesson in life. If your first child is very young, however, he may not even understand the concept of a baby brother or sister, so don't feel frustrated if he doesn't respond as you expect.

Financial considerations

Having a child, as you know, is not cheap. The current costs of a child in the first year are approximately £4,000.00 and there is no doubt that

---

ONLY CHILDREN

Until a second baby arrives, your firstborn is an only child. And if he's aged three or four years and still doesn't have any brothers or sisters, you may be worried that he'll become spoilt, precocious and more comfortable in the company of adults than he is with children his own age. Yet that is not an inevitable outcome. Psychological studies involving thousands of children have found that an only child (when compared to a child with brothers and sisters) is no more likely to be spoilt, attention-seeking or demanding than any other child. Having his parents' love and attention all to himself does not automatically make him selfish – it all depends on how he is managed at home. In fact, an only child often makes a better leader, and frequently shows excellent initiative when required to do so. It seems that mixing mainly with adults during his early years teaches him how to think about others and how to work as part of a team. The evidence from research confirms that an only child is usually just as happy as any other child, and is just as self-confident.

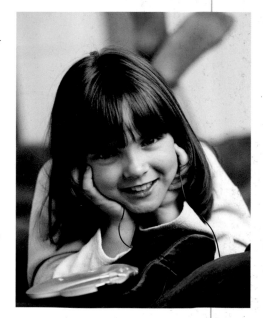

the cost of bringing up two children is greater than bringing up only one – more food, nappies, clothing, extra equipment toys and child care, if you work. Moreover, overcrowded accommodation puts everyone under pressure so if your current home hasn't enough space for a bigger family, you may also have to afford a bigger home as well.

And what about when your children are older – will you be able to afford school fees or university costs? Do you need to work for some time to save money for a second child, etc.?

Practical issues

Situations like manoeuvring a double pushchair down a narrow supermarket aisle, getting two children up the stairs if you live in a two-story home and supervising a toddler while changing a nappy can be quite a challenge. There is also the effect on any travel plans or going back to work.

Managing the routine of two children requires a great deal of planning and unless you are good at organising domestic schedules, this prospect may seem daunting. Even if you have existing arrangements for childcare, these may need to be changed if you have a second child.

On the plus side, however, having spent time raising your first-born child, the chances are that you are more confident about your parenting ability and less anxious than you were the first time round. You have chucked away the parenting L-plates and no longer agonise about the small details that used to trouble you when your first baby was young (like whether he should wear the white jumper or the blue one). And the basic baby-care chores that used to baffle you (such as bathing, changing, dressing) are no longer the huge challenge they once were.

5 tips for making a decision

1 **Make up your own mind** By all means, listen to other peoples' views, but you need to make your decision when it comes to planning for your second.

2 **Avoid over-planning** Life doesn't always go according to plan, and you may not conceive your second child exactly when you want.

3 **Remember there are no guarantees** Although the research suggests some behaviour is associated with each age gap, things can turn out quite differently.

4 **Be positive** Every child is unique, with his own special blend of traits and characteristics. The age gap between siblings is only one influencing factor on personality.

5 **Enjoy your second child** Whether or not the age gap turns out as planned, take as much pleasure from your children as you can.

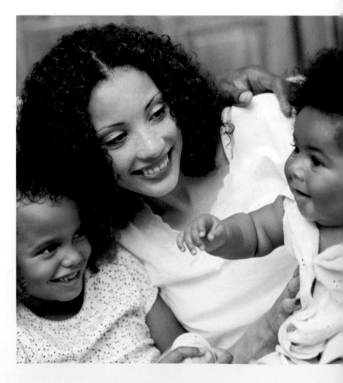

Optimal spacing

Now that you've decided on a second pregnancy, there are again a number of factors – medical, physical, psychological and practical – that will affect when this should happen. Here we consider the timing, while in the next section (see page 12) we look at how and what might happen.

How much time you leave between a first and second pregnancy is influenced by individual factors. This means that a time frame that was best for a friend or your sister might not be best for you. Choosing when to have your second child should be based on you and your partner's unique characteristics and circumstances. You should never be pressured by others into making this decision. There is also your children's perspective to consider. The age gap between your children will have an effect on their relationship with each other, which in turn has an effect on you. If their interactions are positive, everyone in the family benefits; if they are negative, everyone in the family loses out. You also need to think about the impact of a second child on the relationship between you and your partner. However, it's important to realise, that no matter how much you anticipate, no matter how much you weigh up the pros and cons of having a second pregnancy now, there are no guarantees that the new baby will be born exactly when planned!

Medical issues

Interestingly, there are some real medical considerations when it comes to inter-pregnancy interval and the health of both baby and mum.

Studies have shown that the interval between the birth of one child and the conception of the next is one of the factors associated with preterm birth, low birth weight and a baby not growing optimally within the womb. The highest risk of these complications is associated with an interval of less than six months between pregnancies; the least risk is with intervals of 18 and 23 months, with the risk continually increasing after 24 months.

A very short interval between pregnancies may not allow sufficient time for the mother to recover from the physical stresses and nutritional depletions of the previous pregnancy. In addition, for those women who had a caesarean section in the first pregnancy, studies have shown that a short inter-pregnancy interval can increase the risk of uterine rupture if they then attempt a vaginal birth after caesarean (VBAC).

A long inter-pregnancy interval could mean that you are much older this time around and therefore have a higher chance of chromosomal abnormalities. If you are older, there is also a greater likelihood that you are overweight or have developed medical problems that could complicate your pregnancy.

While it isn't always possible to time these things perfectly, it is useful to know what some of the issues are so you can do your best to optimise your situation. For example, you should try to correct any vitamin deficiencies, watch your weight and talk to your doctor about looking out for signs of preterm labour and low birth weight.

Age-gap effects

The difference in ages – whether big or small – will influence you and your children in a number of different ways.

A shorter age gap

If your children will be close together in age and of the same sex, there will be some financial benefits: you may be able to re-use your first child's baby clothes and equipment and your firstborn's toys are probably in good condition as well. You have already adjusted to the reduction in income when number one came along, so the financial impact of having a second child close in age to your first is not as great as when you have returned to work and got used to two incomes once again.

A short age gap also involves minimal disruption to your lifestyle and family rhythms. After all, you and your partner are used to handling a young baby – it's not a distant memory – and you accept that your life revolves around your baby's schedule. You are familiar with having your previous level of personal freedom as a childless couple curtailed in order to meet your baby's needs. so the arrival of a second baby will not result in a dramatic change to your daily routine.

The "down" sides are the additional costs involved and the added pressures on yourself. Looking after two children is more physically demanding than caring for one and in order to cope, you should be in good health and have fully recovered physically from your first pregnancy.

A larger age gap

A gap of more than a few years between your first and second child helps you gain more experience of raising a child, and probably increases your confidence in your parenting skills.

You'll be more adept at managing child care tasks and at organising and maintaining a dynamic daily routine for your children which can only be good news for you and them.

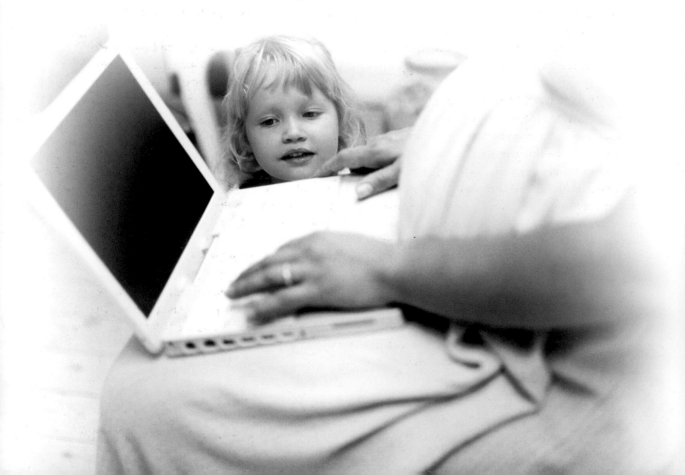

A larger age gap also means that your older child may be at school when the new baby arrives, giving you lots of time with your baby during the day without taking attention away from the older one. And, if sufficiently older, your older child can be a help with a new baby.

Emotional issues

But there are other implications to your children's age gap. If it is two years or less, the chances are that you will not have returned to your career since your first child was born, or perhaps you didn't even have the opportunity to establish a career before you became a parent. As a result, you may harbour feelings of frustration and resentment, which will be reflected in your relationships with your children. A larger age gap will have enabled you to return to the workplace, even if only temporarily, and therefore you may feel more confident about taking time off again for your second child. Your children will sense this positive attitude.

On the other hand, children with a small age gap between them are more likely to grow up as friends because their developmental stages are quite similar. They will know each other very well, and may be better at sharing and playing with each other than when there is a big age gap.

Your children's points of view

When parents have limited time and resources – which is the reality in every family – jealousy can arise between the children.

Known as sibling rivalry, bad feelings occur because the children feel they have to compete with each other to get their fair share of their parents' attention and resources. Sibling rivalry is always unpleasant and is the root of many family squabbles, but there is hardly a family that doesn't experience it at some time or another. It therefore pays to be aware of its relationship to children's ages (see box).

Sibling rivalry may not be immediately apparent. Often, an older child adopts a "wait-and-see" attitude, and it's only when it finally dawns that the new baby is here to stay, that problems arise.

SIBLING RIVALRY

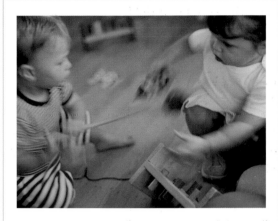

The age gap between children has a direct effect on how likely there will be conflict between siblings. Rivalry is:

Very common when the age gap is between two and four years, because the older child is very aware of the new arrival's presence. He sees the attention showered on the younger sibling and understandably may resent it.

Less common when the age gap between the two children is under two years. Because they are so close in age, they tend to have the same interests, especially when they are older. They are more likely to cooperate than to compete. Sibling rivalry is also less common when the age gap is more than four years. The older child has his own routine, his own friends and his own space by the time his younger sibling is born, which means the baby has less impact on his existing lifestyle.

Almost non-existent when the age gap is 10 years or more. A child aged 10 years or older doesn't feel threatened by the arrival of a new baby in the family. If anything, he is more likely to view this as a positive addition.

Getting pregnant the second time around

It may have been only 10 months since your first child was born, or it may have been five years or more. In any event, you may not remember exactly how to optimise your chances of conceiving or you may be having trouble. The following information provides you with the basics as well at looking at some issues that may have come up in your first pregnancy that can impact on your conceiving.

Obviously if you are reading this book, you have a pretty good idea about how to get pregnant, after all you've done it once before. However, it may have happened really easily the first time, and this time it could take longer (or vice versa). It's important to

realise that there are ways to make the process more efficient so that you can get pregnant as quickly as possible. Efficiency is all about figuring out when you are ovulating (when the egg is being released from the ovary) and getting the sperm to meet up with it at the right time.

Reviewing ovulation

Normally ovulation occurs 14 days before you get your period. If you have a typical 28-day cycle, this will happen on day 14, counting day 1 as the first day of your last period. If your cycle is 32 days long, ovulation should occur around day 18, and if your

MENSTRUAL CYCLE

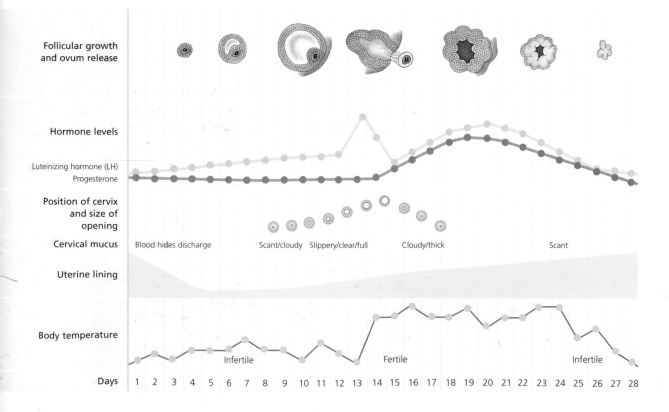

Follicular growth and ovum release		
Hormone levels		
Luteinizing hormone (LH) Progesterone		
Position of cervix and size of opening		
Cervical mucus	Blood hides discharge	Scant/cloudy Slippery/clear/full Cloudy/thick Scant
Uterine lining		
Body temperature	Infertile	Fertile Infertile

Days 1 2 3 4 5 6 7 8 9 10 11 12 13 14 15 16 17 18 19 20 21 22 23 24 25 26 27 28

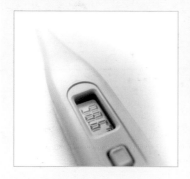

DIGITAL BASAL THERMOMETERS

These thermometers track your basal body temperature for evidence of ovulation. It turns out that your temperature rises close to the time of ovulation. You take your temperature every morning before getting out of bed. It is lowest right before your pituitary gland releases a special hormone called LH (luteinising hormone), which triggers ovulation. Two days after LH is released, your temperature rises about ½ to 1 degree above the baseline. If you get pregnant, it remains elevated and, if not, it falls down to baseline. There are some special thermometers available in chemist shops that actually have a beeper to alert you to the peak temperature reading, which can be really helpful in charting your temperature.

OVULATION PREDICTION KITS

The kits contain test strips that detect the LH hormone (see above) in your urine. When the strip turns positive (in some cases you see a smiley face) it means that you will ovulate within 24 hours.

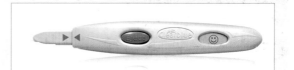

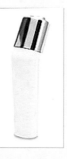

SALIVA FERTILITY MONITORS

When you are about to ovulate, your saliva begins to form a distinctive fern-like pattern when viewed under a microscope, due to an increase in the amount of oestrogen present within the saliva. Kits that monitor your saliva involve you applying a small amount of saliva to a slide and waiting 5 minutes. You then look at the slide under the special microscope and wait for a fern-like pattern to predict ovulation within 24 to 72 hours.

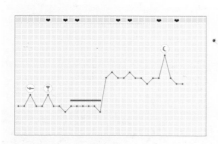

FERTILITY SOFTWARE

"Techies" may like to access fertility software (available on the internet), which helps interpret basal body temperature and cervical mucus to predict your most fertile days. They have colour-coded calendars and each cycle can be charted on a single screen.

cycle length is 25 days in length, it will occur on day 11. Typically, fertilisation of the egg by the sperm will occur within 24 hours from the time it is released, so it's important for you and your partner to manage to get the sperm to reach the egg as soon as possible after ovulation – ideally around 12 to 24 hours later. The best way to achieve this is to try to time intercourse to occur about 12 hours prior to ovulation. That way, the sperm have already made their way up the vagina, cervix and uterus to the fallopian tube where the egg is drifting along towards the uterus. Fertilisation takes place within the fallopian tube, and the fertilised egg makes its way down to the uterus to begin implanting itself within the wall. Sperm are believed to live inside a woman's body for one to two days, although it has happened that they have survived for as long as a week.

Predicting ovulation

When you have a child at home to take care of, you may find that you don't have as much time as you did when you were just a couple for wonderful romance and sex (see chapter 5). Due to time constraints and sometimes sheer physical exhaustion, you may want some help to better predict ovulation, so you can make the most out of the time spent alone with your partner. There are a variety of bodily changes and "tools" available to help predict the moment ovulation should occur (see previous pages).

The effect of age

Clearly when you are having a second (or third or fourth) child, you aren't as young as you were the first time around, even if you feel it! Unfortunately when it comes to fertility, time is not always on your side. It turns out that fertility declines with advancing age – especially after the mid-30s. Don't

HEALTH FIRST	pre-conception issues

If you (or a close relative) had a previous pregnancy involving a neural tube defect (anencephaly, spina bifida) which result from failure of the embryological neural tube to close, it is extremely important for you to be on extra doses of folic acid for at least one month prior to conception. Your doctor should prescribe 4–5 mg of folic acid per day. This will greatly reduce the chances of this problem recurring.

If you had gestational diabetes in your last pregnancy, check whether you were tested with a 75 grams glucose tolerance test at least six weeks after you delivered to ensure that you do not have diabetes when you are not pregnant. If you didn't have that test performed, and you are currently not yet pregnant, you can take the test now. If you are already pregnant, speak to your doctor or midwife about taking the glucose test early to ensure you don't have diabetes.

be too discouraged though, because it has been documented that the oldest woman to conceive naturally was 57 years old, and through IVF, women in their 60s have given birth to healthy babies.

As you get older, the time it takes to achieve getting pregnant can take longer. The chance of getting pregnant on the first try starts to decline in a woman's early 30s, with a more rapid decline by her late 30s. This decline in fertility is probably related to aging of eggs, decreasing number of eggs and a change in the hormonal environment. Also, lifestyle can play an important role: older women may have less frequent intercourse, and are more likely to be obese. These are certainly some factors that may be in your control.

Finding time for you and your partner to be intimate, and getting in the best physical shape possible prior to conception, can be very helpful strategies. If you have been trying to conceive without success, it is worthwhile seeing a fertility specialist after six months (aged 35 and over) to one year (aged under 35). The good news is that there is often plenty the reproductive endocrine and fertility specialists can do to help you achieve a successful pregnancy.

Infertility evaluation and treatment

Some couples find that while they had no problems conceiving the first time around, they experience difficulty getting pregnant again. It's hard to believe, but for many different reasons, over a million couples face "secondary infertility", or problems conceiving after having conceived successful pregnancies previously. This may be related to a long time period between the first and second, or changes in health or lifestyle. The ability of a couple to become pregnant depends on many factors in both men and women. Nearly two-thirds of cases of infertility is due to male and female factors, and the rest is a result of both or is unexplained (see chart). Whatever the reason, the good news is that great strides have been made in helping couples with fertility issues become pregnant, with new and exciting treatments available in the field of infertility and assisted reproductive technology.

Evaluation of infertility in men and women

Fertility in men requires normal functioning glands such as the hypothalamus and pituitary gland as well as normal functioning testes. Evaluation includes taking a thorough history and physical examination, performing an analysis on the semen (sperm count) and sometimes some blood tests.

The evaluation of infertility in women also involves taking a complete history, a physical exam, blood tests for certain hormones such as FSH (follicle stimulating hormone), LH (luteinizing hormone) and prolactin, and tests to evaluate ovulation. Often other tests are performed to evaluate the uterus and fallopian tubes such as a hysterosalpingogram (HSG) where dye is injected into the uterus and an x-ray is taken to see the shape of the uterus and patency of the tubes. Alternatively, hysteroscopy (whereby a small tube with a camera is inserted through the cervix into the uterus to

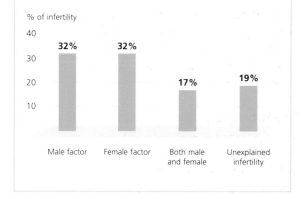

CAUSES OF INFERTILITY BY SEX

Research carried out by the Human Fertilisation and Embryology Authority (HFEA) showed that 32 per cent of the causes of infertility can be attributed to female problems, 32 per cent to male problems and 17 per cent to a combination of both. The remaining 19 per cent falls into a category called unexplained infertility, where a specific problem could not be found in either the man or the woman.

% of infertility

40 — 32% 32% 17% 19%
30
20
10

Male factor | Female factor | Both male and female | Unexplained infertility

actually see tinside the uterus) is performed. Both men and women may be advised to undergo certain tests to check for genetic or chromosomal abnormalities.

Overview of treatment of female infertility

If weight problems – being overweight or underweight – are thought to be a factor, weight modification can help enhance fertility. For problems with ovulation, your doctor may try various medications to help. Clomiphene citrate can help release gonadotropins (hormones such as follicle stimulating hormone, FSH, and luteinizing hormone, LH) to trigger ovulation. Metformin is often used by women with a condition called PCOS (Polycystic ovarian syndrome) to enhance ovulation. Sometimes treatments with gonadotropins themselves, usually in the form of injections under the skin, are helpful in producing many eggs and causing ovulation to occur. Many of these treatments have good success rates, but can lead to a higher incidence of twins and triplets. Sometimes other causes, such as problems with the fallopian tubes, fibroids in the uterus or scarring within the uterus itself, are amenable to surgical treatment.

Overview of treatment of male infertility

Some cases of male infertility are due to problems in the testes, or problems with the transport of sperm from the testes to the urethra through which the sperm are ejaculated. A small percentage is due to conditions involving the pituitary gland or hypothalamus, and many are unexplained. Treatment may involve using gonadotropins, treating genital infections, surgically repairing a

"varicocele" which is a dilated vein like a varicose vein in the scrotum, or even correcting blockages within the male reproductive tract. If a man has undergone a vasectomy in the past, and then changes his mind about having more children, he may undergo a procedure that reverses the vasectomy. Over half of couples can successfully become pregnant after such reversal.

IVF (In Vitro Fertilisation)

IVF is a treatment for infertility in which a woman's eggs are fertilised by sperm outside the body in a laboratory dish. One or more of the fertilised eggs, or embryos, are transferred into the woman's uterus with the aim of producing a pregnancy. With IVF, sometimes the couple trying to achieve pregnancy may use their own eggs and sperm, although sometimes donor eggs or sperm may be used. In other cases, a couple's embryos may be placed into another woman.

Briefly, the process of IVF starts by using fertility medications to increase the number of eggs, or follicles, that develop in the ovaries and to control the time of ovulation. Frequent office visits to measure hormone levels and to perform ultrasound scans to

FACTORS RESPONSIBLE FOR INFERTILITY

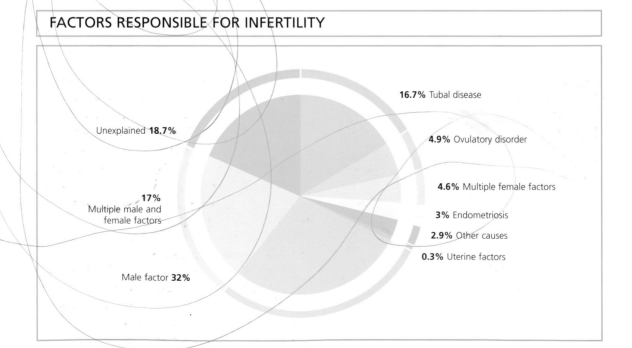

16.7% Tubal disease

Unexplained **18.7%**

4.9% Ovulatory disorder

4.6% Multiple female factors

17%
Multiple male and
female factors

3% Endometriosis

2.9% Other causes

0.3% Uterine factors

Male factor **32%**

IVF MAY BE CONSIDERED IF...

In vitro fertilisation may be carried out when couples have the following issues:
- Severe male factor infertility with very low sperm counts, or abnormal motility or shape of the sperm; in some cases where the male has no sperm, donor sperm may be used
- Absent or blocked fallopian tubes
- Severe endometriosis, after failing with other treatments
- Ovulatory problems not helped by other therapies
- Unexplained infertility, after failing other treatments
- Ovarian failure, where a woman fails to produce enough eggs
- A woman without a uterus, or other medical problems where she should not carry a pregnancy. In this case, a surrogate would be needed

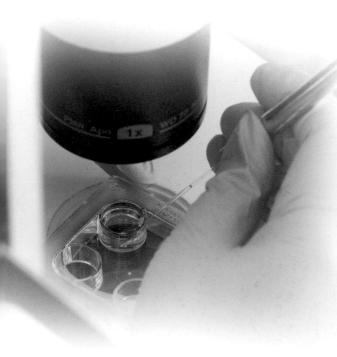

evaluate the ovaries are necessary. A few days after the woman's menstrual cycle begins, a series of injections are started to help the eggs grow within the ovaries. At some point, an injection of hCG (human chorionic gonadotropin) is given to trigger ovulation. Usually the eggs, or follicles, will be ready to be retrieved with 36 hours. The egg retrieval involves using a needle to withdraw the egg from each follicle through the vagina, under ultrasound guidance. The eggs are then brought to the lab, where they are combined with sperm within a dish. In general, about half of the eggs will become fertilised. In some cases of male infertility, a special procedure called ICSI (intracytoplasmic sperm injection) will also be performed where the sperm is injected directly into the mature egg. Then about two to five days after retrieval, one or more fertilised eggs, or embryos, will be placed into the woman's uterus through a thin tube inserted directly through the cervix. The number of eggs transferred depends on the quality of the embryos, the woman's age, the couple's preferences, the previous history of pregnancy and miscarriage and the number of prior IVF cycles. About two weeks after the embryo transfer, a blood or urine test for hCG, the pregnancy hormone, can be performed to see if pregnancy has occurred.

Preimplantation genetic testing and diagnosis

If you had prior pregnancies affected by either certain chromosomal abnormalities or genetic diseases, and want to keep this from happening again, you may be a candidate for IVF and preimplantation genetic diagnosis (PGD). This refers to a technique in which one or two cells from an embryo achieved through IVF is removed and tested. PGD is an alternative to the usual way of testing for certain chromosomal or genetic diseases after pregnancy is achieved by conventional methods such as amniocentesis or chorionic villus sampling (CVS). The advantage is that it allows only embryos to be transferred that are not affected by affected by a specific condition. Disadvantages are that PGD requires that a couple undergo IVF to conceive, and that many other conditions are not detected by PGD.

Choosing the sex of the baby

Maybe you already have a son at home, and you are hoping to have a little girl to balance things out? Or maybe, you have a daughter, and are hoping you can give her a younger sister to play with? There are several different reasons, both personal and even medical, where couples may desire to control the sex of their next child. And whether or not they want to influence gender, most couples (over 90 per cent) would like to know the sex of their expected child before the birth.

The most common reasons for gender selection include a personal preference for a child of a specific gender to achieve a family "balance" with children of both genders, to avoid certain genetic disorders that involve the sex chromosomes or to avoid certain diseases more common in a particular sex.

Whatever the reason, there are certain methods that are used, with variable success rates, to help couples achieve their goals (although gender selection based on personal preference is not available in the UK). The only treatment with a 100 per cent success rate (at least in determining gender) is PGD – though it is an invasive and expensive procedure.

The sex of a child depends on whether the X-containing egg is fertilised by a sperm bearing an X or Y chromosome. Most of the "natural" methods are based on influencing the environment within the vagina so that it becomes more receptive to X- or Y-bearing sperm. As well as diet and timed intercourse, various sexual positions, are said to be likely to produce a girl rather than a boy (and vice versa).

Diet
The "Preconception Gender Diet" is based on the theory that a couple can improve their chances of having a baby girl by increasing their dietary intake of

DID YOU KNOW...

Sex selection
Attempts to influence the gender of offspring have been around since ancient Egyptian time. Even Aristotle got in on the act by giving advice on certain sexual positions to achieve boys or girls.

calcium and magnesium. To improve chances of a boy, they should take in more sodium and potassium. Little follow-up data is available to confirm whether this works.

Timed intercourse
The idea behind timed intercourse is the belief that Y-bearing sperm swim faster, but do not survive as long, as X-bearing sperm. There isn't any good data to support that timing works in gender selection.

Sperm sorting
In this case, semen is separated into X and Y bearing sperm by a variety of methods. Y-bearing sperm have smaller heads, greater swimming ability and a lower negative charge than X-bearing sperm. Sperm carrying the desired gender is used for fertilisation by either intrauterine insemination or IVF. There are many different techniques that are used, with variable results. One specific technique (PGD) sorts sperm by the amount of genetic material. X-bearing sperm are 2.8 per cent heavier than Y-bearing sperm, which forms the basis for the sorting technique. Success rates for achieving the desired gender are about 93 per cent for females and 82 per cent for male. Long-term data are needed to confirm the safety and effectiveness of this technique.

PGD (Pre-implantation genetic diagnosis)
In couples undergoing IVF, PGD, as discussed above and on page 19, can be used to identify male or female embryos, and only embryos of the desired gender would be introduced into the uterus. Rarely errors in gender determination can occur.

2

SAME, SAME, BUT DIFFERENT

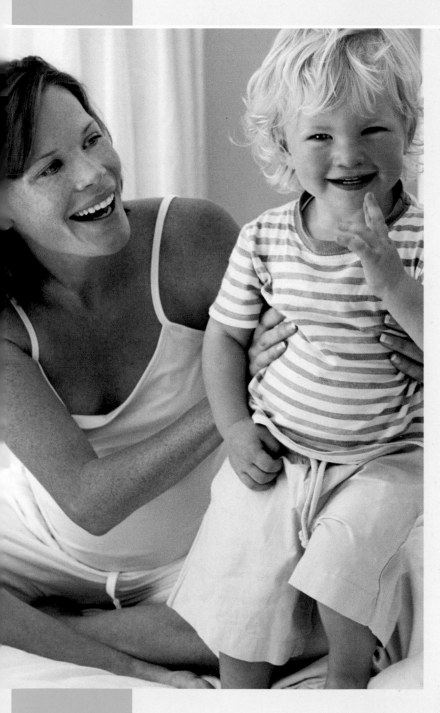

There are no hard and fast rules when it comes to second pregnancies. Some things may be very similar to the first time around, while others are totally different. Recognising that you are carrying a completely different baby, and may experience completely different symptoms should make you feel relieved if things don't go exactly as they did the first time around. If you had terrible morning sickness the first time, and few bouts of nausea this time around, consider yourself lucky! That being said, there are some common and unifying scenarios that women having their second baby experience.

Physical considerations

Fatigue

If you are wondering why you can barely get through the day without trying to catch a quick nap, put up your feet for a few minutes or find that you can't stay awake past 8 p.m. at night, you are not alone. Many women having their second baby feel an overwhelming sense of fatigue, particularly in the first and third trimesters. It is not quite clear why it seems to be worse the second time, but one explanation may be that you don't have the luxury of only taking care of yourself when you are home…you have your other child to look after! While in your first pregnancy you may have come home from a busy day, put your feet up and relaxed on the sofa with a nice book or film, now you are busy playing with your firstborn, giving baths, cooking dinner and putting him to bed. Also, you may find that you don't have the time to exercise and eat well, both of which can help to give you some more energy. So here are some tips: don't hesitate to ask for help when you are feeling tired, so you can get the rest you need. Try to keep some healthy snacks around to munch on, and if possible, get some exercise (even walking is useful) to keep your energy levels up!

Showing earlier

We have patients who ask us all the time how it is possible at only 10 or 12 weeks to be already finding their clothes too small. At this time, the uterus is still within the pelvis and it should be too early to be "showing". However, it is really quite common for women to look four months pregnant at this time, but not because the uterus is larger but because the abdominal wall muscles are more stretched out and lax from the previous pregnancy. Early on in pregnancy, the elevated progesterone

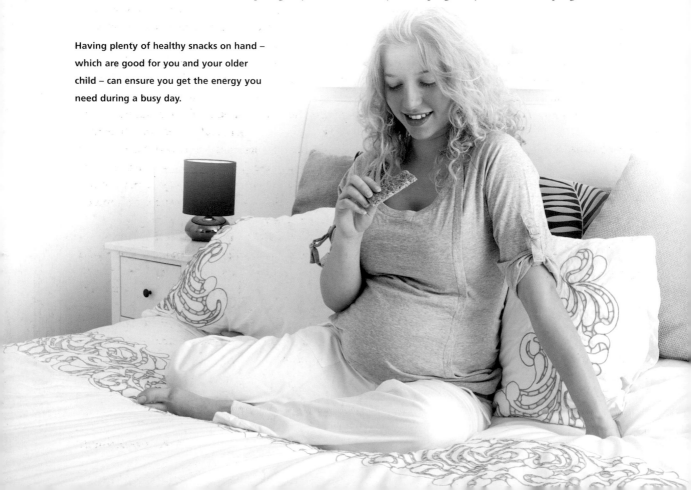

Having plenty of healthy snacks on hand – which are good for you and your older child – can ensure you get the energy you need during a busy day.

levels in the blood cause the muscles of the gastrointestinal tract (stomach, bowels) to slow down. This then leads to some abdominal distention, bloating and constipation, and the more relaxed muscles of the abdominal wall can't keep everything hidden as well. The result is that your bowels make your stomach protrude more, and you look like you are showing much earlier!

Breast changes

Among the first symptoms you may notice are soreness, tenderness and sensitivity in your breasts. Having experienced them once before, they may be the first sign to alert you to the fact that you are pregnant. Some women experience more tenderness and enlargement, while others experience less. Other common changes are an increase in breast size, bluish streaks across the breasts (which are really just enlarged blood vessels), sore and itchy nipples and occasionally a throbbing pain. While some women experience more tenderness and enlargement, others experience less the second or third time around. Diminished symptoms are often associated with previous breastfeeding.

If you aren't so lucky and find that you are pretty uncomfortable, consider wearing cotton-only bras, make sure you have a bra that is supportive and the right size for you, and try putting cold compresses on your breasts if they feel very hot and itchy.

Stretch marks

Medically known as striae gravidarum, stretch marks occur in over 50 per cent of all pregnant women. They usually occur on the abdomen, but can occur on the buttocks, thighs and breasts – really any location where the skin is being stretched. Stretch marks usually start out pink in colour, but over time turn silvery-white. If you were lucky enough to avoid getting them the first time, there is a good chance you won't get them the second time around. If you, like many women, did get those "battle scars" of pregnancy, you may be predisposed to getting them again. Either way, there are some things you can do to lessen your chances of getting them again or for the first time.

Because stretch marks may be more common with greater weight gain, keep your eye on your weight to avoid excess weight gain and try to exercise to maintain good muscle tone.

There are some creams, which may be effective in helping to reduce the development of stretch marks. Two creams have been studied scientifically and showed a reduction in their formation. One study used massage with a cream called trofolastin, which contained centella asiatica extract, alpha tocopherol and collagen-elastin hydrolysates, while the other used massage with an ointment containing tocopherol, panthenol, hyaluronic acid, elastin and menthol. (A search on the internet may be necessary to locate the creams.) Some women have also tried using vitamin E but the effectiveness of this is unclear. If you find that your stretch marks are particularly bothersome, consider seeing a dermatologist a few months after you deliver.

Varicose veins

Varicose veins are those annoying, bluish-coloured worm-like looking bulges that seem to grow under the skin of your legs, and sometimes even thighs. They are dilated blood vessels that have become enlarged because of pressure from the growing uterus on the major blood vessel that returns blood to the heartthe inferior vena cava. As if this weren't enough, the greater amount of blood and fluid within the blood vessels, and the relaxing effect that the progesterone has on the veins adds further to the formation of these dilated veins. If you managed to escape varicose veins the first time, you may not be so lucky the next. They tend to increase with more pregnancies, as well as with age.

There are some things that you can do to decrease the chance of getting them. Try to put your feet up whenever you can, and try to force yourself to wear support stockings, especially elastic stockings found in surgical supply stores that require a prescription from your doctor. These stockings can do wonders at preventing the development of varicose veins.

Pressure in the vaginal area

One of the most common complaints of women having their second baby is about the tremendous pressure they feel in the vaginal area and the lower pelvis. This usually starts around 20 weeks, and continues through most of the pregnancy. Women are usually concerned that the pressure is not normal, and they are most worried about premature labour. However, rest assured, this is usually just the sensation of pressure of the enlarging uterus. No one knows for sure why women feel this so much more the second time around, but most likely it is due to more relaxation of both the abdominal and pelvic floor muscles.

Fetal movements

Most women find that they feel fetal movement a lot earlier than the first time around – often at four months. This may be due to the fact that they know just what to expect. With your first baby, you may not have been sure whether the movement was really the baby or just gas pains. Now that you know what it really feels like, you are more likely to notice it earlier. If you don't feel it early, though, don't worry because there are other factors involved in how well you feel movement. Sometimes when the placenta is implanted on the anterior surface of the uterus, or the surface closest to your abdomen, it is harder to feel the baby's movements.

Braxton-Hicks contractions

That tightening you feel across the uterus that is noticeable, but not painful, known as Braxton-Hicks contractions, tends to be more frequent and starts earlier in a second pregnancy. Some women feel this as early as the late second trimester. It's also pretty common for them to be more painful in the third trimester. You may even think that you might be in labour! A lot of women feel that they should "know" when they are in labour the second time around, but often it's not that clear. Don't be embarrassed if you call your caregiver thinking that you are in labour when really you are just having strong Braxton-Hicks contractions. Even women having their sixth or seventh child are not always sure!

Stress incontinence

It may have happened a few times during the last pregnancy, and for some time after delivery of their first child, but now you may find that you leak urine when you laugh, cough or sneeze on a more regular basis. The relaxation of the pelvic floor muscles and the weakening of the muscles from the delivery of your first child are partly responsible for this situation. Being pregnant again, with the added pressure of the uterus on the bladder can aggravate the situation.

If this truly becomes a major problem, take frequent trips to the bathroom to empty your bladder on a regular basis. Also, practising Kegel exercises, which are designed to strengthen the pelvic muscles, can help; often things do get better after the delivery.

PELVIC MUSCLES

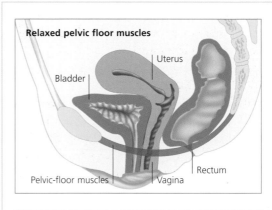

Relaxed pelvic floor muscles

Uterus

Bladder

Pelvic-floor muscles

Vagina

Rectum

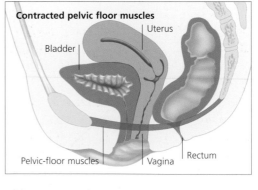

Contracted pelvic floor muscles

Uterus

Bladder

Pelvic-floor muscles

Vagina

Rectum

Emotional considerations

A feeling of achievement

Although you're an "old hand" at getting pregnant – you managed to conceive the first time or you wouldn't be waiting for your next – you'll probably still have a terrific sense of achievement when you discover that you are pregnant for a second time. This feeling of elation will be even stronger if conception took longer than expected. Most mothers assume that if they became pregnant as planned the first time round, the same will happen the next time. But life doesn't always go according to plan. For a whole raft of reasons (see page 17), the second pregnancy could be more difficult to achieve. That's why you should be proud of your achievement, whether your second pregnancy was timed exactly as you wanted or whether it took so long that you began to wonder if you would ever get pregnant again. Pregnancy can never be taken for granted. Your family life is about to change yet again in so many wonderful ways.

Accepting baby's gender

Attitudes to baby gender vary, especially the second time. When you had no children, you probably had a mild preference for a boy or a girl – that's only natural – though the chances are that you'd have been happy with whatever you got, as long as your baby was healthy. But the position may have changed slightly this time. After all, you already have a baby of one gender at home and you could be thinking that one of the opposite sex would be a good balance. And, of course, there are some parents who for whatever reason have a very definite preference (see also page 20).

There's nothing wrong with gender preference, as long as it doesn't get in the way of your parenting. Each newborn baby – boy or girl – has the same emotional needs to be loved, and to feel valued, safe and secure. Bear in mind that your baby didn't choose his or her gender. The problem with allowing yourself to develop a very strong and obvious desire to have a baby of particular gender from your second pregnancy is that this is likely to have a negative effect in the long run.

Think about it. If you invest a lot emotionally in having, say, a boy this time because you had a girl the last time, your extreme reaction at a son's arrival could easily put your first-born girl's nose out of joint. Hearing you talk about how important having a boy may reduce her self-esteem and make her feel less important to you. Likewise, if you don't deliver a baby of the gender you hope for, your enthusiasm for your second one could drop dramatically. Either way, someone loses out when gender expectation becomes too dominant.

Adjusting to inevitable changes

No matter how well prepared you are for the arrival of your second baby, no matter how confident you are in your parenting skills having gained experience from looking after your first child, there are a number of further changes in family life that can have a powerful emotional effect.

To start with, there's the financial impact. It is said that "two are no more expensive than one" but that's simply not always the case. You'll have one extra mouth to feed, there will be increased energy bills because you'll be at home for longer periods and eventually the stream of hand-me-downs from baby number one will begin to lessen (older children tend to wear through their clothes quicker than babies), especially if your children are not the same gender. Add the other ingredient of reduced family income because you are now not working again (if you managed to return to work at all after your first baby), and you have a recipe for financial pressure that could easily put you under stress.

Have realistic expectations. Accept that for a while – maybe even for only six months or a year if you plan to return to work and use childcare for your two – money will be tight. There will be less for the luxuries of life. But so what? This is only a small temporary price to pay for the delight of having a growing family. Saving as much as you can between baby number one and two also helps cushion the economic blow. Surveys consistently show that the most common cause of fights between parents is money – do what you can to make sure that you and your partner are an exception.

Coping with time pressures

Then there are changes to family routines. You have probably just managed to get your life into manageable shape, as a parent caring for a young baby. The initial shock to the system has passed and you have developed coping skills that you never even knew existed beforehand! And now that everything is ticking along nicely, thank you very much, a further sea change is about to occur. The physical demands of childcare chores for two is more demanding than for one. Don't worry, though – you'll soon feel that you are in control.

Give yourself time to adjust, and get as much help from your partner as you can. Apart from breastfeeding, there is no babycare task that is the exclusive domain of either mum or dad (even with breastfeeding, mum can express milk so that her partner can give a feed later while she rests). Forward planning of the day's activities will be extremely helpful.

Loving two as much as one

The most common fear of parents who have one child and are now expecting their second is that they won't love the second as much as the first (or vice versa). So if this thought is running through your head right now, rest assured that you are not alone. You have such a close attachment with your existing child that it's hard to imagine loving another one as well. After all, you can't believe that another child could be as terrific as the special individual who already occupies pride of place in your family.

But you will love your second child as much as you do your first. You may love this child in different ways because he or she will have different strengths and weakness, but it will be parental love all the same. The fact is that all parents have the capacity to love lots more children than one. Mother Nature wouldn't have given women the ability to have many children if the ability to love them all wasn't inbuilt as well. You'll respond with love to your new baby as you become acquainted with his or her personality and adapt naturally to this baby's needs, just as you did with your first baby. It may help to recall that there were times before your first child was born, when you were anxious that life with three of you at home would be very different from life with just you and your partner, and you worried that you would never adjust to parenthood. Yet very quickly life with three seemed totally normal. The same will happen when your second comes along (and your third…). All you need to do is to relax and go with the flow. Be yourself – that's who your second baby wants to get to know. You'll find you are just as able to form a strong emotional connection with baby number two as you have with baby number one.

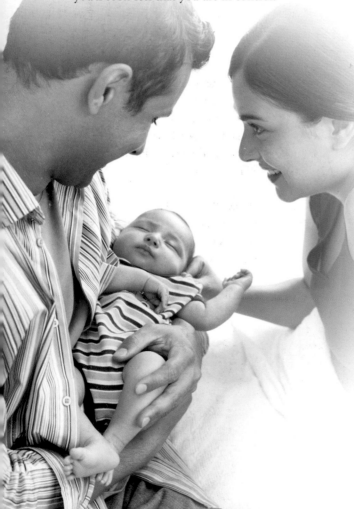

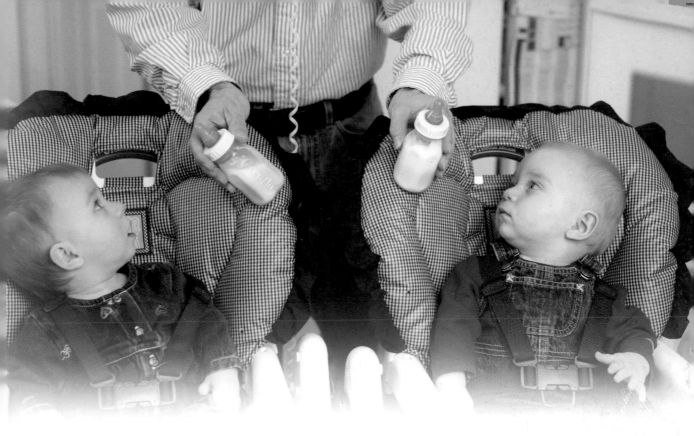

Parenting twins

Twins bring twice as much delight and excitement to parents, but they also bring twice as much work. Managing the daily routine of two young children is demanding enough, managing that routine for three takes it to another level altogether. If you are having twins at your second delivery, don't panic.

Ask for help, and accept it when offered. The practicalities of feeding, changing, bathing and dressing two babies the same age at the same time, with an older child who also needs attention, is challenging for even the most competent parent. That's why you should be prepared to look for support, whether from your partner, from relatives or from friends. And if you are lucky enough to receive spontaneous offers of help, take them. That doesn't mean you can't manage on your own, it's simply a very practical solution to help you juggle the continuous babycare demands.

You'll feel a lot happier and a lot less stressed about developing a special relationship with all your children if you make a particular effort to give individual time to each of them. Time is tight when you have two young babies to look after at the same time. You'll probably spend the bulk of your time just working through the daily chores, which will leave you with little time left for anything else. Whatever time you have during the day, however, it will be worth trying hard to spend some moments alone with each twin rather than spending time only with the two together.

Having confidence in yourself

No matter what worries you have about coping with the emotional impact of a second baby, bear in mind that you already have a good track record. You have learned a great deal about yourself since those early days of your first pregnancy; you have also learned new caring and management skills. That's the solid emotional foundation which you will bring to raising your second child and why you can be confident you'll cope with all the psychological stresses and strains that raising two children might bring.

Key decisions

Prior to your baby's birth, you may need to make certain decisions that can affect both you and your baby. If you are expecting a baby boy, you may need to decide if he is to be circumcised. Due to technological advances, it has recently become possible to save and store your baby's cord blood, and this is something you may want to do.

Circumcision

Removing the foreskin – the skin at the end of the shaft of the penis that covers the glans, or head of the penis – has been practised since Biblical times. Religious Jews traditionally have the procedure performed when a boy is eight days old. Many Muslims circumcise their boys at an older age.

Studies have shown that a boy's chance of getting a urinary tract infection is slightly lower following the procedure. Circumcised males have a lower risk of acquiring HIV infection following intercourse with an unprotected HIV-positive partner. Other sexually transmitted diseases are also less likely in a circumcised male. The same is true for cancer of the

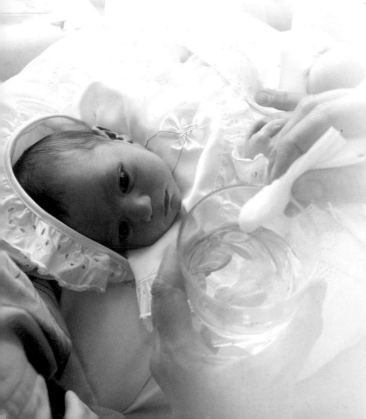

head of the penis. Another benefit of this procedure is that care of the glans is easier and hygiene is improved. Phimosis, or sticking of the under surface of the foreskin to the glans, which can be uncomfortable, is avoided.

On the other hand, there are those who believe circumcision is a painful and unnecessary practice. Urinary tract infections aren't very common in boys and cancer of the glans is exceedingly rare. Cleaning of the glans is not so difficult. When a boy is two or three years old, the foreskin will readily retract to allow proper hygienic care. Phimosis is not that common and is readily treated. In rare cases, bleeding and infection can result.

Circumcision has a few benefits and a few complications. It is uncomfortable, but not that bad when anaesthesia is used. Since the points in favour of and against its use are relatively closely balanced, you should do whatever seems best to you. If the ease of caring for the glans or the reduction in uncommon infections holds high value to you, choose circumcision. Likewise, if there are religious reasons, it's a family custom or if you feel your son will otherwise be different from his peers, the procedure seems a reasonable choice. On the other hand, if the discomfort and chance of remote but serious complications hold sway, then avoid it. You also may want to consider what your son will think about it when he is older.

Storing cord blood

The blood in your baby's umbilical cord contains stem cells made by your baby, which have the potential to differentiate into many kinds of blood cells or organ tissues (muscle, liver, etc.). Should she ever need a bone marrow (or possibly other organ) transplant, your child's stem cells will be a perfect match; there is no risk of rejection by the body's immune system and medications given to suppress the immune system in hopes of preventing rejection would not be needed. Stem cells can be grown in cell

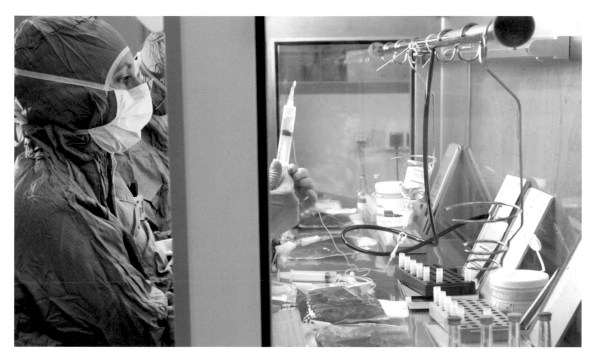

Laboratory which is storing and conditioning cord blood.

culture artificially or can be stored in a frozen state for later use.

If your hospital allows the procedure, stem cells from cord blood can be obtained at the time of delivery. A kit from the storage facility with receptacles for the cord blood is required, but you can obtain it weeks before your delivery by contacting the cord blood bank you plan on using. They will charge a fee for their services. After the umbilical cord is cut, your doctor or midwife will insert a needle into the umbilical vein and withdraw blood for storage. The blood comes from the umbilical cord and placenta when it is no longer attached to your baby; it is not taken from your baby. If you chose not to store cord blood, there is no use for this remaining placental blood and it is discarded.

Although growing in popularity, storing cord blood is not without problems; some children who go on to develop leukaemia already have pre-leukaemic cells in their cord blood, which can reinfect them. In the UK, NHS cord blood banks are public ones; they store donated blood for use by patients anywhere in the world who need a

DID YOU KNOW...

Checking your records
If your first pregnancy was not straightforward, or you want to know more about what happened during the birth, you might want to see your maternity notes. Write to the data controller of the Medical Records Department at the hospital in which your baby was born. Ask the hospital to send the notes plus copies of all attached documents, such as letters and laboratory results sheets. There may be a charge for this.

transplant. Private banks, which are generally located in the US, are for-profit organisations, which store cord blood for possible future use by an individual's own family for a fee. All UK-based banks must comply with the EU Cells and Tissue Directive, enforced by the Human Tissue Authority and Medicines and Health Regulatory Agency.

Common second pregnancy myths

If this pregnancy is different from your first, it means that the sex of your baby is also different from the first.

So many women think that if they were nauseous the first time around and had a boy and aren't nauseous the second time, they must be having a girl. Same thing with developing acne, fatigue carrying differently. None of these differences correlate with having a baby of a different gender.

I can't get pregnant because I'm breastfeeding.

If you are reading this book before becoming pregnant, bear in mind that while the chance of getting pregnant is less while breastfeeding, it is NOT zero. Pregnancies definitely do happen while breastfeeding. The hormone, prolactin, which stimulates milk production, can also decrease the chances of ovulation occurring. But every woman is different, and hormone levels vary. Some women's ovaries continue to release eggs despite the secretion of prolactin.

If you are reading this book because you are pregnant for the second time, and conceived while breastfeeding, you know first hand that the idea that breastfeeding prevents pregnancies is false.

Neither is it true that you have to stop breastfeeding when you are pregnant (see also pages 72 and 73).

I can skip many of my antenatal visits because my first pregnancy was uncomplicated.

While hopefully your second pregnancy will be just as perfect, it is still important to see your caregiver regularly. New situations can arise that weren't an issue the first time. For example, some women develop gestational diabetes in a second pregnancy, even though they didn't have it the first time. In addition, urine and blood pressure checks and talking about symptoms are important features of antenatal visits in every pregnancy.

If you conceived when your first child was awake your children will fight all the time.

Well, we can tell you this is completely untrue. First of all, how many of you know if your firstborn was asleep or awake at the moment of conception? Anyway, almost all siblings will fight at some point so don't blame yourself for finding the time for romance whenever you can.

If your first child is a terrible sleeper, your second one will be a great sleeper.

Again we wish we could guarantee you plenty of restful nights, but there isn't any good predictor of how well and soon a newborn will sleep through the night. Establishing a routine sometimes is useful, but babies, to some degree. have minds of their own and will sleep on their own schedule. If you are really experiencing difficulty getting your child to sleep through the night, don't hesitate to talk to your GP or health visitor. Meanwhile, try getting as much rest as possible before the arrival of your second child.

Second babies are always bigger.

While it is true your second baby might be bigger than your firstborn – plenty of second babies are the same size or smaller than their siblings. In a second pregnancy, you're more prone to developing gestational diabetes, which can make your baby bigger, and you may have gained weight since your first pregnancy, and heavier women tend to have heavier babies. On the other hand, in a second pregnancy you're less likely to develop pre-eclampsia, which can cause your baby to be smaller.

3

ANTENATAL CARE

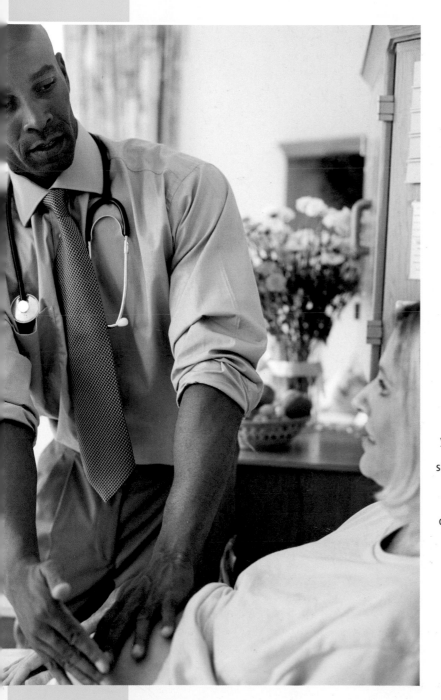

The first time you found out you were pregnant, you probably rushed to the phone to schedule an appointment with your doctor as soon as possible. This is pretty normal for excited first-time mums. The second time around, women tend to be a little more laid back and seek antenatal care later than they did with their first pregnancy. Don't wait too long though, because it is important to see your doctor early so that he or she can establish your due date accurately, which is is best done during the first trimester.

Visits

If your first pregnancy progressed normally, your schedule of antenatal visits will be similar the second time around, although you will probably be seen less frequently. If there were complications in your first pregnancy, however, your doctor or midwife may see you more frequently in your second pregnancy, depending on the nature of the complications. For example, if you developed blood pressure problems with your first pregnancy, your caregiver may see you more often towards the end of the second trimester. As a general guide, the chart on the opposite page shows the main antenatal appointments usually offered to women who have already had a baby with no problems during the pregnancy, and the timing of the key tests offered. Changes to this schedule may occur if you are expecting more than one baby, are diabetic or you have some other underlying medical condition (see also page 34).

Where you'll be seen for your checks and tests, depends somewhat on your choice of caregiver (see page 34). If you work with an independent midwife, she'll carry out most of your antenatal checks at home with tests done in hospital. Otherwise, your GP and community midwife will provide most of your antenatal care, probably in the doctor's surgery, and you will go to the hospital for scans and diagnostic tests, if necessary. If your care is linked to a midwife unit, you will be looked after during pregnancy by a team of midwives.

If you have a pre-existing medical problem, you may have regular checks with a hospital-based consultant and all care may be carried out in hospital. There are some conditions such as heart conditions which may require the care of two specialists; an expert in the medical condition as well as an obstetrician (a doctor who specialises in maternity care).

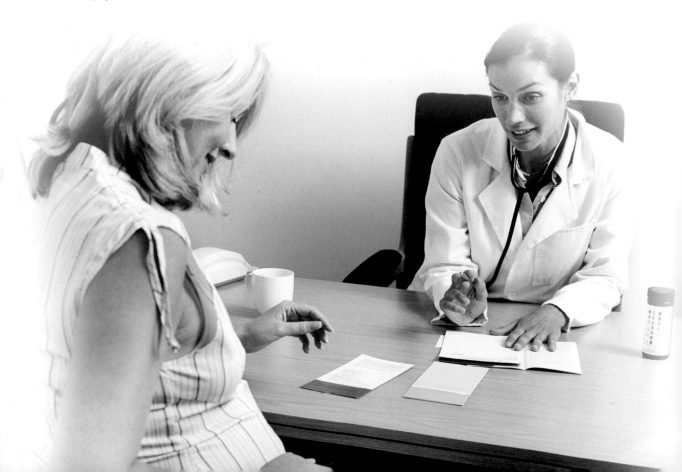

SCHEDULE OF ANTENATAL APPOINTMENTS AND TESTS

In a second pregnancy there are generally seven basic appointments, although the number and timing of appointments may vary depending on the centre you visit and your individual circumstances. In addition, hospital visits will be necessary for certain tests.

10 weeks	Booking appointment, which includes discussion of medical and lifestyle issues, baseline blood tests and discussion of possible screening tests
10–14 weeks	Ultrasound scan to determine gestational age
10–13 weeks	Chorionic villus sampling (CVS)
11–14 weeks	Nuchal translucency screening
15+ weeks	Amniocentesis
15–20 weeks	Blood tests to hellp assess the risk of Down's syndrome
16 weeks	Follow-up appointment to include discussion of results, blood pressure, and urine check
18–20 weeks	Anomaly scan to check for structural abnormalities
28 weeks	To include blood pressure, urine check, measuring of the fundal height (distance between pubic bone and top of the uterus to assess the size of the uterus and fetus) and blood tests if required
34 weeks	Similar to assessment at 28 weeks, but there may be discussion of pain relief and the birthing plan
36 weeks	To include blood pressure, urine check and assessment of fundal height. The baby's position is checked. Also, discussion may include breastfeeding and issues following delivery, such as care of the newborn and screening tests for the new baby.
38 weeks	To include blood pressure, urine check and assessment of fundal height. Discussion of what happens if go past due date.
40 weeks	Similar to the 38 week appointment

Choice of caregiver

For your second birth, you may be thinking of having a different experience than the first time around, and this may necessitate you choosing a new caregiver. Possibly, you've moved to the UK from abroad or after a hospital delivery, you are contemplating a home birth.

If you decide you want your baby to be born in a hospital, the choice is between a unit, which is part of a large general hospital or a smaller community hospital, or a completely separate NHS or private unit, which is linked to a hospital (in case specialist care is needed). In all cases, your GP needs to arrange a referral. A midwife-led unit offers what is sometimes called one-to-one, domino or team midwifery care. Such a unit may provide midwives skilled in the deliveries of specific groups of women such as high-risk women, young mums or diabetics.

If, after a discussion with your doctor, you are considered a candidate for a home birth (see page 85), you will want to find a midwife who will provide much of your antenatal care and deliver you at home. Some hospitals and midwife units will provide midwives for a home delivery. It is also possible (if expensive) for a woman to see an independent midwife. It is also possible to see a consultant on a private basis.

Tailored treatment

Antenatal care with the second pregnancy will be similar in some ways to your first pregnancy and different in others. Just how different, will depend in large part on three things: the length of time between your first and second pregnancies, the outcome of your first pregnancy and any changes in your health since your first pregnancy.

The greater the lapse of time since your first pregnancy, the greater the changes, as new technology and scientific information becomes available. Most of the routine tests done in the early part of pregnancy haven't changed that much over the years. For example, testing your FBC (your full blood count, which tests for anaemia, among other things) and blood type have been used for decades and are not likely to change. From time to time,

however, doctors add new tests or change old tests that help them improve the outcome for your pregnancies (see pages 40-44).

If you developed complications during your first pregnancy, like preterm labour or pre-clampsia, your doctor will probably change your antenatal care plan. If you've developed medical problems since your first pregnancy, like high blood pressure or diabetes, then you will also need a different plan of care as you will if you are expecting twins.

Antenatal care for older mums

Many women having their second (or third, or fourth...) baby will still be relatively young. Some, however, will be significantly older the second time around. Women over the age of 35 are considered to be of "advanced maternal age". The main issue with age is that the older you are when you conceive, the greater the likelihood of having a baby with a chromosomal abnormality like Down's syndrome. The risk starts to go up at age 30 but increases more rapidly after age 35. This means that you may be more inclined to undergo special tests, such as amniocentesis, that look for chromosomal abnormalities.

If you're healthy and have no medical problems, your antenatal care as an older mum is essentially the same as for a younger woman. If, however, you've developed medical problems like high blood pressure or diabetes, you may have more appointments and extra tests. It is also likely that you'll be recommended to see a doctor for some or all of your appointments rather than a midwife.

Even healthy older mums have a slightly higher risk of pregnancy complications like miscarriage, pre-clampsia, deep vein thrombosis and gestational diabetes. They also have a higher risk of delivering prematurely and needing a caesarean section. These are additional reasons why your doctor or midwife may alter your schedule for antenatal care.

Expecting twins

If you're pregnant with two babies, you will require more than the standard seven antenatal appointments and the two ultrasound scans (see page 38). A multiple pregnancy is considered to be higher risk and it is usual for a consultant to provide the antenatal care. Depending on your medical circumstances, you will, in all likelihood, be asked to attend your consultant's clinic for a monthly check-up while, at the same time, seeing your midwife every four weeks in between – in effect, a visit every two weeks. If you also have an

Age	Risk of Down's syndrome
25	1:1500
30	1:900
35	1:350
40	1:100
44	1:30

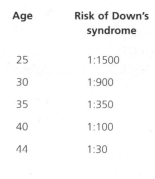

existing condition such as diabetes or epilepsy, you will be seen more often by your consultant and midwife in order to ensure everything is all right with you and your babies.

If you conceived your babies through IVF (see page 18), your consultant may wish to see you more often.

You should also have more frequent ultrasound scans in your last trimester to check the growth and position of your babies.

It is very important to attend all your appointments, so that checks on your blood pressure and urine can be carried out to rule out any possibility of pre-eclampsia, diabetes and anaemia.

Your care may differ depending on whether you are carrying identical or non-identical twins. If your babies share both inner and outer membranes and a single placenta (monochorionic, monoamniotic twins), you can expect increased scans and monitoring. This is because there is a greater risk of a serious problem – twin-to-twin transfusion syndrome (TTTS) – which can cause one baby to grow at the expense of the other

If your babies are identical but have separate membranes and placentas, or are non-identical twins formed from separate eggs, the risks of problems are lower. Twins generally are more likely to be born prematurely; 37 weeks is considered full term for a twin pregnancy, but many women do reach 40 weeks or more. If your babies go overdue, your consultant may suggest induction of labour.

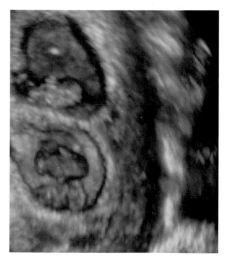

On the left is an ultrasound of a triplet pregnancy. Monochorionic twins, lying in one chorion and amniotic sac and sharing a single placenta are on the bottom, their sibling with his own sac and placenta is on top.

Pregnant women over 40 and those with the following conditions:

- Cardiac disease, including hypertension
- Renal disease
- Endocrine disorders or diabetes requiring insulin
- Psychiatric disorders (being treated with medication)
- Haematological disorders
- Autoimmune disorders
- Epilepsy requiring anticonvulsant drugs
- Malignant disease
- Severe asthma
- Use of recreational drugs such as heroin, cocaine (including crack cocaine) and ecstasy
- HIV or HBV infection
- Obesity (body mass index 30 kg/m$_2$ or above at first contact) or underweight (body mass index below 18 kg/m$_2$ at first contact)
- Women who smoke
- Women who are particularly vulnerable or who lack social support.

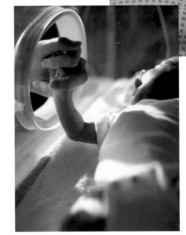

Women who have experienced any of the following in previous pregnancies:

- Recurrent miscarriage (three or more consecutive pregnancy losses or a mid-trimester loss)
- Preterm birth
- Severe pre-eclampsia, haemolytic anaemia, elevated liver enzymes, and low platelet count (HELLP syndrome) or eclampsia
- Rhesus isoimmunisation or other significant blood group antibodies
- Uterine surgery including caesarean section, myomectomy or cone biopsy
- Antenatal or postpartum haemorrhage on two occasions
- Puerperal psychosis
- Grand multiparity (more than six pregnancies)
- A stillbirth or neonatal death
- A small-for-gestational-age infant (below 5th centile)
- A large-for-gestational-age infant (above 95th centile)
- A baby weighing below 2.5 kg or above 4.5 kg
- A baby with a congenital abnormality (structural or chromosomal).

Ultrasound scanning

Ultrasound technology uses a small hand-held transducer to generate ultrasound waves so named because they are outside of the hearing range of the human ear. The ultrasound waves pass through your abdominal then uterine walls and are reflected off of your developing baby. The reflected sound waves are processed by a computer to generate an image of the baby. Since the image is constantly being updated, you can also see your baby moving around inside your womb. Some of the sound waves can also pass inside your baby, allowing you to see the developing organs and structures.

There are many types of ultrasound examinations (also called sonograms or scans) that your doctor may recommend during your pregnancy. Most women these days have at least two ultrasound exams, but this depends on your doctor or midwife's preferences and your personal history – expecting twins, for example, you may need several scans.

The anomaly scan is a comprehensive examination of your baby from head to toe to evaluate the developing organs and structures. The scan is typically done between 18 and 20 weeks gestation because by that time, the fetal structures are big enough to be seen clearly using the ultrasound waves.

Ultrasound technology is constantly improving so don't be surprised if things look different the second time around. Now, many congenital abnormalities can be diagnosed earlier. For that reason, some doctors will recommend that you undergo an early anomaly scan between 14 to 18 weeks. This doesn't replace the routine scan, though, because some of the structures at an early anomaly examination have not developed clearly enough to evaluate them properly. Often, it is possible to tell whether a baby is a boy or a girl during the early scan, but this is almost always possible by the routine anomaly scan.

Types of scan

There are routine ultrasounds and those that may be carried out in special situations.

Routine scans

A dating ultrasound is usually done in the first trimester at around 10 to 14 weeks and, as the name suggests, is used to help date the pregnancy (to tell exactly how far along you are) and to establish your most accurate estimated due date (EDD). During the scan, the crown-to-rump length (the length from the top of the embryo's head to its tail end) is measured to determine gestational age. If this exceeds 84 mm, the head circumference is used. In addition to establishing your EDD, you can see on the scan your embryo's heart beating on the scan, which confirms that the pregnancy is viable.

The nuchal translucency scan of the space behind the fetal neck is part of the first trimester screen (see page 40) and is generally done between 11 and 14 weeks of pregnancy.

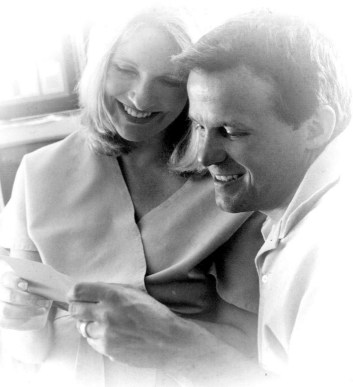

A growth scan may be done at around 32 weeks of pregnancy to make sure that a baby isn't growing too big or too small. The ultrasound technician may measure different parts of the baby and puts the measurements into an equation generating an estimated fetal weight (EFW).

The EFW can be plotted on a graph to compare your baby to other babies at the same gestational age to see what percentile it comes in at. The average for any given gestational age is the 50th centile, but anywhere between the 10th and 90th centile is considered appropriate for gestational age. Above the 90th centile is considered large-for-gestational age (LGA) and below the 10th centile is considered small-for-gestational age (SGA).

If your doctor or midwife thinks that your baby is growing as it should, you probably won't have a growth scan. However, if you had growth problems with your previous pregnancy or if you are carrying twins, your doctor may recommend that you have these periodically throughout the second half of your pregnancy.

The ultrasound examinations described above are considered routine, although your doctor may not recommend that you need to have all of them, depending on your individual circumstances and what happened in your first pregnancy.

Non-routine ultrasounds

Issues may arise during your pregnancy, which your doctor may want to evaluate with an ultrasound. Reasons for having an ultrasound exam include:
- bleeding or spotting;
- not feeling the baby move regularly;
- to check the amount of amniotic fluid.

If you had a premature birth in your previous pregnancy or if your cervix started to open early, your doctor may recommend that you undergo periodic transvaginal ultrasounds (the ultrasound transducer is placed gently inside the vagina) to check the length and appearance of the cervix.

If your baby isn't growing as well as it should, your doctor may recommend a type of ultrasound known as a biophysical profile (BPP). This test is usually done in the third trimester and is essentially a "check-up" on the baby to make sure it is still doing fine inside the womb. The technician assigns points for fluid and the baby's movement patterns.

ASSESSMENTS AT THE ANOMALY SCAN

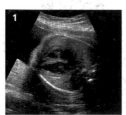 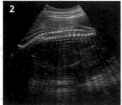 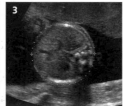 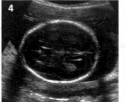 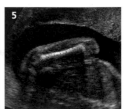

During this scan, the ultrasound technician will want to check on all the organs of the body and take some useful measurements.

When the heart is visualised (1), the ultrasound technician will check to see that it is occupying about a third of the chest and points to the left; that there are four chambers, which are equal in size; and that the major arteries are connected correctly.

The spine (2) will be examined to ensure that the posterior spinous process is present along its length in order to rule out neural tube defects.

Baseline measurements will be taken of the abdominal circumference (3) head circumference (4), and the length of a femur, one of the leg bones (5).

If the baby scores high enough, both you and your doctor can be reassured that the baby is OK to stay inside the womb for a while longer.

The most recent advance in ultrasound technology is 3-Dimensional and 4-Dimensional ultrasound. This amazing technology is changing on an almost daily basis and may not have been available for your first pregnancy (and it still isn't used on a routine basis for every pregnancy). Traditional ultrasound utilises 2-D technology and provides flat images or pictures. 3-D technology, as the name implies, shows the baby in a 3-D picture format. 4-D ultrasound is similar to 3-D but is visualised in real-time, meaning that you can see your baby moving during the ultrasound. Doctors are finding more and more ways to use this technology, usually to help clarify uncertainties on regular 2-D scans, but some day, 3-D and 4-D technology may replace traditional 2-D technology.

Doppler ultrasounds show uterine artery flow and can help doctors assess problems such as slow growth in the fetus and high blood pressure in the mother.

Are they safe?

Many mums ask: "Are all of these ultrasounds safe for me and the baby?" Ultrasound technology for medicine has been around since the 1960s and numerous studies have shown that it is safe for both babies and mums. Since it involves only sound waves, there is no radiation involved, so you don't have to worry about that, as you do with x-rays. The latest ultrasound machines are designed so that the person doing the scan can use the least amount of energy needed to visualise the baby.

The benefits of ultrasound are numerous. In addition to reassurance that everything is normal, some abnormalities can be treated while the baby is still in the uterus and even for the ones that are diagnosed but can't be treated before the birth, it is important to know before birth so that the appropriate treatments are lined up in a timely fashion after the birth.

So, in experienced hands, ultrasound is safe and will provide numerous benefits to you and your baby.

DIFFERENT TYPES OF SCANS

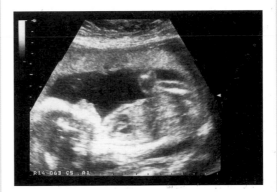

2-D ultrasound

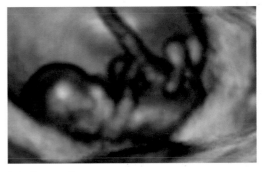

3-D ultrasound

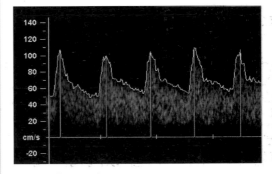

Doppler ultrasound

As well as helping doctors to assess how well your baby is developing, ultrasound scans of various types also reassure parents and help them to bond with their new offspring. Seeing their baby usually makes parents feel more relaxed and less fearful about the outcome.

Diagnosing abnormalities

The main screening tests offered on the NHS are the "combined test" between 11 and 14 weeks, and for women who book late in pregnancy the "triple" or the "quadruple", or "quad", test between 15 and 20 weeks. Other tests may be available in certain areas or privately. The results of the screening tests are used, together with the gestation of the pregnancy and the maternal age, to calculate the chance of having a baby with Down's syndrome.

There are two approaches commonly used to help detect chromosomal abnromalities. Screening tests are used to help refine your baseline (age-related) risk for having a chromosomal abnormality. Diagnostic tests (sometimes called "invasive" tests), on the other hand, allow specialists to examine the chromosomes and can tell you with almost 100 per cent certainty whether they are normal or not.

Screening tests use ultrasound measurements, measurements of certain substances in your blood, or both to generate a risk estimate for your baby having a chromosomal abnormality. If your risk is above a certain threshold, then your doctor will recommend that you undergo a diagnostic test to get a definitive answer about the chromosomes.

The downside to screening tests is that they will miss a small percentage of babies with chromosomal abnormalities. The downside to a diagnostic test is that it is invasive and carries a small chance of causing a miscarriage.

Screening tests

The first trimester screen is usually done between 11 and 14 weeks. It involves using ultrasound to measure the nuchal translucency (NT), which is a space behind the fetal neck, and a blood sample to measure hCG (a hormone) and PAPP-A (a substance produced by the placenta). The first trimester screen will detect about 80 to 90 per cent of babies with Down's syndrome. There are several ways that you can get your results, depending on your wishes and your doctor's preferences.

Together these tests are known as the "combined test". You get the results within a few days of having

NUCHAL TRANSLUCENCY AND NASAL BONE LENGTH

During the first trimester screening ultrasound, the fluid-filled area or nuchal translucency (1) behind the baby's neck (boxed), is measured. A computer programme is then able to give each mother an individualised risk assessment for Down's syndrome in the fetus based on the mother's age and the size of the nuchal translucency in the fetus.

The presence of a nasal bone has recently proven to be an early and good marker for assessing the risk of Down's syndrome. If, during the first trimester screen, ultrasound examination shows that a nose bone (2) is present, the risk of Down's syndrome is reduced by a factor of three.

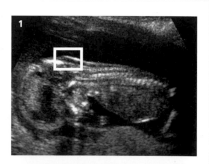

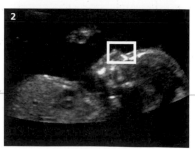

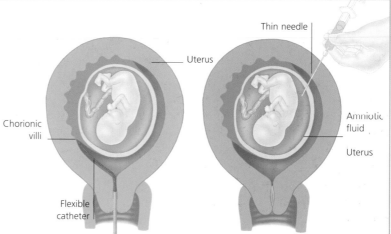

CVS (left) and Amniocentesis (right) are both diagnostic tests that can be carried out if an abnormality is suspected. Amniocentis is more commonly used than CVS as there is less risk to the baby. With both tests ultrasound is used to guide the doctor to the right location in the uterus and to avoid injury to the baby.

the tests done, usually still within the first trimester. If the results indicate that your risk for a chromosomal abnormality is increased, then you have the option of a chorionic villus sampling (CVS) to check the chromosomes.

In the "integrated test" you do everything that you do for the combined test, but you don't get your results right away. You come back between 15 and 20 weeks to have your blood taken again for a second trimester "triple" or "quad" screen (see below). The laboratory will integrate the results of the combined test and the second trimester screen to give you a single result. If the results indicate that your risk for a chromosomal abnormality is increased, your doctor will advise you about having an amniocentesis. The advantage of this test is that it has a slightly higher Down's syndrome detection rate and is less likely to suggest that Down's syndrome is present when it is not.

If you didn't make it to your doctor or midwife early enough to get scheduled for a first trimester test (or if you don't want one), you can still have a second trimester screening test between 15 and 20 weeks – the "triple test", which measures three blood components to generate a risk assessment for Down's syndrome or the "quad test", which measures four substances (AFP or alpha-fetoprotein; hCG or human chorionic gonadotropin; uE3 or unconugated estriol and INH-A or inhibin-A).

The Down's syndrome detection rate with the quad test is pretty good and ranges from 75 to 80 per cent. If you have had a combined test alone or if you had a CVS (see below), you won't need the whole quad test. You will only need the AFP part of the test because in addition to playing a part in diagnosing chromosomal abnormalities, AFP is also important in helping to diagnose neural tube defects like spina bifida and other fetal defects.

Diagnostic tests

Some women may want to forego the screening tests and go directly to a diagnostic test. The two diagnostic tests commonly available are amniocentesis and chorionic villus sampling (CVS).

Amniocentesis

Amniocentesis is typically done between 15 and 20 weeks of pregnancy. Using ultrasound, a doctor will guide a small needle into the amniotic cavity in an area away from the baby and remove about 20-30 milliliters (about 2 tablespoons) of amniotic fluid. The cells in this fluid are cultured in the laboratory for several days then stained with special stains so the chromosomes can be analysed and a karyotype (a picture of the individual's set of chromosomes) produced. On average, it takes about seven to 14 days to get the final results.

It used to be thought that the risk of having a miscarriage after an aminocentesis was as high as 0.5-1 per cent (1 in 200 to 1 in 100). Recent studies have indicated, however, that the risk is probably much lower – in the range of 1 in 1,000.

Chorionic villus sampling

Commonly known as CVS, chorionic villus sampling is another diagnostic test used to check for chromosomal abnormalities. It is typically done earlier than amniocentesis – between weeks 10 and 13 of pregnancy. CVS has been around since the mid-1980s but has recently become more and more popular because of the first trimester screening mentioned above. If a woman finds out from her combined test at 11 weeks, for example, that her baby is at an increased risk for having a chromosomal abnormality, she can have a CVS at that time to find out definitely, rather than waiting anxiously for an amniocentesis at 15 to 20 weeks. Also, if a chromosomal abnormality is, indeed, confirmed and she decides not to continue the pregnancy, termination can be carried out earlier in the pregnancy, which may be less distressing.

CVS can be done in one of two ways – either transabdominally or transcervically. The transabdominal approach is very similar to amniocentesis. Using ultrasound, the doctor guides a small needle into the developing placenta (instead of the amniotic cavity as is done with amniocentesis), where the chorionic villi are located. The cells in the chorionic villi came from the fertilized egg, so they contain the same chromosomes as the developing baby. A few of the villi are removed and sent to the lab for analysis.

The karyotype you get from a CVS is essentially the same as the one you get from amniocentesis. So, if you have a CVS, you don't need an amniocentesis later on (except in very rare circumstances, which are outside of the scope of this book.)

The second way to do a CVS is transcervically. With this approach, the doctor places a speculum in the vagina to hold back the vaginal walls so the cervix (the opening to the womb) can be seen. The ultrasound technician holds the ultrasound transducer on the abdomen to show the doctor

where the placenta is located. The doctor then passes a tiny flexible plastic catheter through the cervix into the placenta, and removes a few of the chorionic villi.

The decision to have a transabdominal or transcervical CVS is based on two factors. The first is the location of the placenta. Often, the placenta will be positioned within the uterus in a way that it is easier to get to via one way rather than the other. The second consideration is the experience and training of the doctor. Some doctors have only been trained in one technique or prefer one to the other.

Since amniocentesis (and CVS) are invasive procedures, they carry a small risk of causing a miscarriage. It is unclear why this risk exists. Many people think it is caused by introducing infection into the uterus, but we now know that this is not always the case. Others think that it is related to the experience of the doctor performing the test. Although experience is important, even the most experienced of doctors will see miscarriages after these procedures. Most doctors used to quote a miscarriage rate after amniocentesis of about 0.5-1 per cent (1 in 200 to 1 in 100). These figures came from studies that were done in the 1970s and early 1980s – over 25 years ago. Many doctors always felt that this miscarriage rate was an overestimate and not what they were seeing in their day-to-day practice. Also, ultrasound technology has improved dramatically over the past several decades enabling doctors to see the developing baby and surrounding structures more clearly, so it only makes sense that the accuracy of placing the needle has also improved. Recently, several studies have indicated that the risk of miscarriage after an amniocentesis is probably closer to 1 in 1,000 – much lower than previously thought.

It was also previously believed (and some people still believe) that CVS is riskier than amniocentesis. Studies done in the last few years comparing the two procedures, however, have shown that there is no statistical difference between miscarriage rates after amniocentesis and those after CVS. The decision about which procedure to undergo, if any, should be made after a careful discussion of the options with your doctor.

Genetic testing

Genetic testing may be arranged during pregnancy, Since your genes don't change, you may think that you don't need to go through this sort of testing in your second pregnancy if you had genetic tests in your first. With genetic disorders like cystic fibrosis, if you were found not to be a carrier in the first pregnancy, then you don't need to repeat the test in your second pregnancy. But some disorders require further testing in subsequent pregnancies and new tests are constantly being developed to test for other disorders, so you may need to be tested with each pregnancy.

Tests are now available to diagnose Fragile X Disease and Spinomuscular Atrophy (SMA). Fragile X Disease is an inherited cause of severe learning difficulties. It affects about 1 in 4,000 males and 1 in 8,000 females. Anyone with a family history of this disorder or of severe learning difficulties where a cause hasn't been diagnosed should be tested to see if he or she is a carrier for fragile X. Individuals with developmental delay or autism can sometimes have fragile X. If you have someone in your family with one of these disorders, ideally, that person should be tested to see if they carry the gene first, but your doctor may order the test directly for you in order to save time.

SMA is a severe neuromuscular disorder that affects about 1 in 10,000 births. It is called a "recessive" disorder, which means that both partners in a couple have to carry the gene for any of their children to inherit it. Carrier testing for this disorder is now available, however, the test will only detect about 90 per cent of people who carry an SMA-causing gene.

New tests

Chromosomal abnormalities make up the majority of inherited abnormalities in developing embryos. Certain other genetic disorders, like cystic fibrosis and Fragile X disease mentioned above, are not so uncommon. As scientists identify more of the genetic mutations that underly particular disorders, new tests for less common genetic disorders are being developed.

SCREENING FOR GENETIC DISORDERS

There are a group of abnormalities that are more common in individuals of Ashkenazi (eastern European) Jewish descent. The individual disorders themselves, even though they are more common in that group of people, are still pretty rare – ranging from about 1 in 1,000 to 1 in 50,000, depending on the disorder. In order for a couple to have a child with one of the disorders, they both have to carry the gene for that disorder. Carrier screening is available for some of these genetic disorders and others are frequently being added to the list, as new tests are developed. If you have a family history of one of these disorders, you should consider being tested. Also of note, even if only one partner is an Ashkenazi Jew, screening may still be recommended for that individual.

- Tay-Sachs Disease
- Canavan Disease
- Fanconi Anaemia (Group C)
- Gaucher Disease
- Glycogen Storage Disease

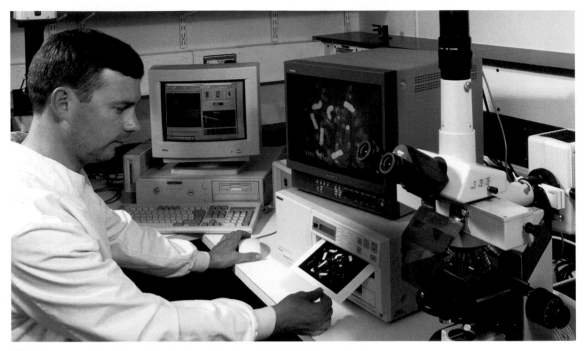

FISH (fluorescence in-situ hybridisation) is a technique that highlights a particular gene or chromosome so it can be checked for abnormalities.

A panel of tests for a group of disorders called "microdeletion syndromes" has recently been developed. These disorders are called microdeletion syndromes because they are caused by the deletion of a piece of DNA (which makes up the genetic code) that is too small to be seen on a standard karyotype. These disorders are relative rare – occuring anywhere from 1 in 1,500 to 1 in 50,000 newborns. The testing uses FISH technology. FISH stands for fluorescent in situ hybridisation, which describes the scientific way of doing the test. The cells in this fluid are cultured in the laboratory for several days then stained with special stains so that the chromosomes can be analysed. On average, it takes about seven to 14 days to get the final results. You may, therefore, hear the doctor refer to the testing as a "microdeletion FISH panel". Currently, there are about eight disorders included in the panel, but it is anticipated that more will be added as the technology becomes available. This testing isn't considered routine, however, so talk to your doctor to see if it is something worth pursuing for you.

The very latest test to be developed is sometimes called a "microarray test" or "array-based CGH" (which stands for comparative genomic hybridisation – the technique used to perform the test). This test uses the latest technology to check for roughly 150+ genetic alterations that doctors have identified through recent research (the microdeletion syndromes mentioned above are usually included in this test).

A tiny amount of DNA is placed on a small "chip" – much like the chips currently being used in computers. If the DNA being tested has one of the abnormalities coded on the chip, a chemical reaction occurs that causes the chip to change colour in the area on the chip corresponding to the abnormality. A special scanner can pick up the colour change and identify the abnormality. The advantage of this type of testing is that you can test for many different disorders with a very small amount of DNA. Some of the disadvantages are that the technology is very labour intensive and the cost is high.

4

TAKING CARE OF YOUR BODY AND BABY

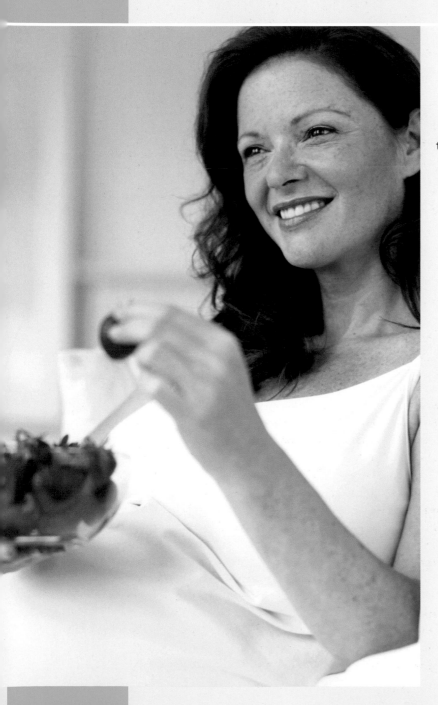

With one child to look after and another on the way, you will need to keep yourself in the best health possible to give your developing baby the start he requires. Key to this will be the common ground between your existing child's and partner's needs and your own – finding healthy foods that will suit the whole family and exercise that fits easily into your daily routine together. You should also take the opportunity to rest and relax when you can.

Your pregnancy diet

Now you are pregnant for the second time, not only will you need to increase the amounts of particular vitamins and minerals in your daily diet, but also ensure you include foods that provide sustained energy rather than quick sugar hits. You will need real stamina to care for your child while pregnant with your second baby.

You may find that smaller and more frequent meals suit you during pregnancy, particularly in the later months as your bump gets bigger. If you have a young child, she will probably have a mid-morning and mid-afternoon snack and this pattern of eating every few hours should work for you both.

What you need

In order to nourish yourself, your developing baby and your existing child, you should put a variety of healthy foods on the table including:

Plenty of fruit and vegetables

At least five portions a day. Remember, they do not always have to be fresh. You can go for other options, such as frozen, dried and tinned.

A varied selection of fruit and vegetables should already be a normal part of your child's diet if she's to establish a healthy eating pattern for life. Cut-up vegetables and fruit, like apples, carrots, and bananas make excellent and convenient finger foods.

Pure vegetable juices and fruit juices (as long as they are 100 per cent fruit and don't contain added sugar) count towards your daily total and there are many available.

Lots of grain-based carbohydrates

Like bread, cereals, pasta, rice and potatoes. These should make up (with fruit and vegetables), the majority of what you eat. Bear in mind that wholegrain is best for you, but not for your child if she is under five. She should have more of the simple grain-based foods like white pasta and white bread.

Protein foods

Important for healthy growth and development. Good sources include meat, chicken and fish (two portions of fish a week, one oily) as well as eggs, beans and lentils. Some types of fish should not be eaten or only in moderation, however, (see page 52).

Dairy foods that are rich in calcium

Calcium is vital for the healthy development of your baby's bones and teeth and the same is true for your growing child. Calcium may also help to prevent high blood pressure Reduced-fat milk, yogurts and hard cheeses made from pasteurised milk like Cheddar and Parmesan or soft cheeses like mozarella

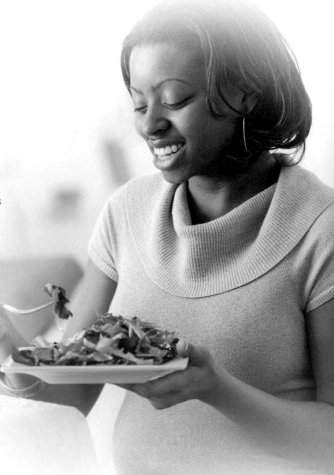

and cottage cheese, fromage frais and crème fraîche are the best choices.

Sufficient fibre

Keep constipation – a common problem in pregnancy and childhood – at bay with plenty of fruit and vegetables. Other good sources include wholegrain bread and pasta (though these should be limited in the under fives' diet.) Drinking plenty of water in combination with a fibre-rich diet will help you to avoid it.

Healthy fluids

Water, milk, vegetable juices, fruit juices and fruit teas are best. Try to avoid caffeinated drinks (see page 52). Aim to drink at least eight 225-ml (8-oz) glasses of fluids every day.

Only a little fat and sugar

Eat minimum amounts of saturated fats (butter, lard, margarine and shortening) and sugars (chocolate, sweets and cakes) because they are high in calories that are essentially "empty." They give you an energy burst, but it's never too long before you feel the need for another. You will need healthy energy-givers that keep you going for the long haul – dried fruit, a piece of malt loaf or a yoghurt. Eating too many sugary and fatty foods or fried foods will also mean you put weight on rapidly rather than achieving the healthy gradual increase you are aiming for. "Good" fats are unsaturated and sources include avocados, fish, nuts and olives as well as olive, vegetable and corn oils.

You should also offer your child the same types of healthy snacks that are good for you. Avoiding chocolates and other

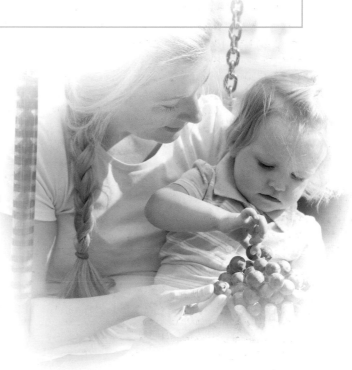

MORE **ABOUT** | the under fives diet

Young children can't manage too much very high fibre food, such as brown rice and wholewheat pasta. These foods can upset their tummies and affect how well their gut absorbs nutrients from the food they eat. This may make them feel tired and even affect their growth. Less commonly, the absorption of important nutrients such as calcium and iron may be affected. In general, young children should eat mainly white bread, rice and pasta with small amounts of wholemeal pasta and bread plus plenty of fruit and vegetables. As your child gets older you can increase the very high fibre foods, but make sure that you don't give her too much saturated fat (in cakes, biscuits, fatty meat and butter).

sugary foods will help set the pattern for her healthy future. A child's eating patterns and preferences are established early in life, so now while she is young, is the time to eat healthily so you both benefit.

Having said all that, there is no need to deny yourself completely. The odd treat is fine.

Special requirements in pregnancy

Ideally, you should be able to get all the nutrients you need from your healthy, balanced diet. However, this is not the case in pregnancy. Two vitamins supplements are recommended for all pregnant women – folic acid (a B vitamin) and vitamin D. It also will be worth talking to your doctor or midwife about taking other vitamin supplements, if you are suffering with morning sickness, suffer from anaemia, are a strict vegetarian or are expecting twins (see also page 85).

Calories

Pregnancy is not a time for dieting and unless you have a BMI (body mass index) over 27, you will probably need to increase your calorie intake in the

GOING ORGANIC

Recent food scares have made buying organic an attractive choice for pregnant women. Many feel the generally higher prices are justified by the fewer chemicals – pesticides, fertilisers, colourants and preservatives – they contain. Some people feel that limiting exposure to additives in the uterus reduces the risk of babies subsequently developing allergic reactions such as asthma, eczema or food allergies. Moreover, organically grown fruits and vegetables may have slightly higher levels of vitamin C, and other important antioxidant substances such as phenols and anthocyanins, which help protect the body and boost the immune system.

If buying all organic is not within your budget, then limit your organic foods to those you eat in the largest quantities – dairy products including milk, fruit and vegetables, for example.

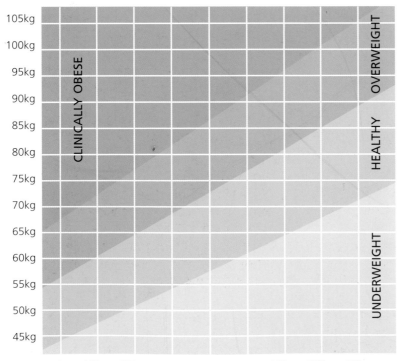

BMI Readings

Body mass index is calculated by taking your weight in kilograms (kg) dividing by your height in metres (m) then dividing the result by your height in metres (m) again. The totals equate as follows:

up to 19 = underweight
20-26 = healthy
27 and over = overweight
30 or more = clinically obese

later months of your pregnancy. How many calories you need depends on your activity levels. Generally, most women need 1800 to 2100 per day, with an increase of around 200 calories a day in the last three months and another increase of 200 calories once you start breastfeeding.

Folate

Folic acid has been shown to reduce the risk of spina bifida and other neural tube defects. It is prescribed as a supplement (see below), but it is worth remembering to include foods in your diet that are rich in folate (a B vitamin), the naturally occurring form of folic acid. These include green leafy vegetables, bananas, brown rice and bread, and cereal fortified with folic acid.

Iron

Some women have iron deficiency in pregnancy so it is worth including iron-rich foods in your diet. These include lean red meat, green vegetables and pulses. As iron supplements can cause constipation, it is better to include some iron-rich foods in your diet. Vitamin C can help the body to absorb iron so you should havie some citrus fruit or juice when you eat these foods. Coffee and tea may reduce the absorption of iron and so it is a good idea to cut down on these (see also page 53).

Calcium

This mineral is needed for the healthy development of many parts of the body including bones and teeth, muscles, nerves and the heart. Good sources include milk, yogurt and cottage cheese, which are favourites with young children.

You will be fine with semi-skimmed milk (and yogurt), but if your child is aged under two, she should have full-fat milk.

Non-dairy sources of calcium include sardines, soybeans, fortified cereal and spinach.

Vitamins

Taking folic acid has been shown to reduce the risk of spina bifida and other neural tube defects. It is recommended that women take a dose of 400mcg

BREASTFEEDING NEEDS

If you are pregnant and breastfeeding, you should eat approximately 500 more calories a day (instead of the extra 200 normally recommended during pregnancy). These additional calories should be particularly nutrient-dense as your breastfeeding diet will need to include 20-50% more of most required vitamins and minerals. Fat consumption is a key component of a healthy breastfeeding diet. A growing baby relies on a variety of fats to be strong and vigorous and breast milk is particularly high in fats retrieved from your diet. Your goal should be to consume 30% of your calories in the form of monounsaturated, polyunsaturated and essential fatty acids. The best sources can be easily found in canola, olive and other vegetable oils along with cow's milk and dairy foods. Meat is also important, but for your own health reasons, choose lean cuts over excessively greasy, red meat.

Water is also imperative for your body and milk supply. Keep a measured cup or bottle with you and drink when your baby does. Make sure you consume at least eight cups of fluid every day.

Being pregnant will change the taste and appearance of your milk – it will take on a colostrum-like composition, be more watery and less white. While these variations do not affect the nutritional value of your milk, your older baby may not like the different taste and texture. For your new baby's sake, try to eat a variety of food flavours as these transmit directly into your breast milk. Research has shown that breastfed babies are extra receptive to a variety of tastes as they grow whereas formula fed babies who eat the same flavours daily tend to resist new foods.

OVERCOMING NAUSEA

Now, with one child to look after already, morning sickness may be even more difficult to cope with than the first time round. No one knows exactly what causes morning sickness, but hormonal changes, tiredness and an increased sense of smell probably play a part. Here are a few ideas to try:

- **Have small, frequent meals** as you may find these easier to cope with. Make every mouthful count by ensuring meals and snacks are packed with nutrients for you and your developing baby.
- **Eat simple foods and avoid spicy meals** A simple ginger biscuit (ginger is often recommended as a remedy for nausea) and hot water with lemon can make a good snack. Try avoiding curries and other hot foods, also fried foods, which tend to cause nausea. You may find eating a couple of plain crackers before you get up in the morning helps to relieve your symptoms.
- **Spend time in the fresh air** Get out as often as possible. This will benefit you and your child.

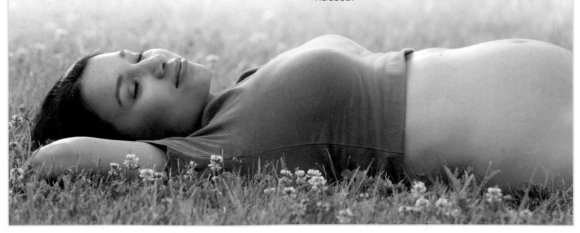

- **Rest when you can** Tiredness may play a part in causing morning sickness. Also, make sure you allow yourself plenty of time to sleep at night.
- **Get up slowly** Give yourself as much time as possible in the morning. Rushing around may worsen your nausea.
- **Avoid getting too warm;** feeling overheated may be a cause.
- **Try to avoid strong smells** open the windows when you are cooking.
- **Eat what you fancy** You need to restrict sugary foods to some extent, but eating what you feel like can sometimes help.
- **Eat protein-rich snacks** Try lean meat, nuts and eggs.
- **Drink water throughout the day** but in frequent small amounts.
- **Try ginger tea.**
- **Never miss meals** Hunger can contribute to nausea.

per day when trying to conceive and, once pregnant, for the first 12 weeks of pregnancy. The recommended dose is higher if you are a diabetic or have had a baby with a neural tube defect. It is a good idea to include foods that contain folate (natural folic acid) in your diet.

The other necessary supplement is vitamin D (10mcg per day) for healthy bones and teeth. It is found in a few foods – oily fish, egg yolk, fortified margarine and spreads. Sunlight helps you to produce it, so build up your supply by spending some time outdoors in clement weather.

As for your child, it is often recommended that children should have supplements of vitamins A and D from six months of age unless they are having more than 500mls of infant formula per day. It is worth discussing whether you child needs them with your doctor or health visitor.

If you do decide to supplement your diet or your child's with added vitamins, it is important to take only supplements that are appropriate for pregnancy or for your child's age.

Expecting twins or more

Although there are no specific guidelines in the UK for nutrition for twin or multiple pregnancies, it is generally accepted that there is a need for additional calories and nutrients throughout the pregnancy. In fact, gaining adequate weight in the first 20 weeks predicts a higher birth weight for the babies. The US Institute of Medicine recommends that regardless of pre-pregnancy weight women pregnant with twins need to gain between 16 and 20 kg (35-45 lbs). Some of this – say 2.5 kg (5 lb) – should be in the first trimester, with a weight gain of 0.7 kg (1.5 lb) a week after this. If you are expecting triplets, you may need to gain a total of around 23 kg (50 lb), or 0.7 kg (1.5 lb) per week.

It is not just additional calories that you require. To support the additional increase in blood volume and your growing uterus as well as the development of two or more babies, you also require additional calcium, essential fatty acids and iron.

It is important that your diet contains a good mix of nutrient-rich foods and an all-round antenatal

NOT FOR THE UNDER FIVES

While you are thinking about which foods are safe for you, you will also need to remember that there are a number of foods that are not suitable for young children. These include:

- **Whole or chopped nuts** they may cause choking. Talk to your doctor before giving your toddler peanuts if she has an allergic condition like allergic eczema or a food allergy (or if parents or siblings have allergies) as she may have a higher risk of peanut allergy. If you do give your child peanuts you should wait until she is six months old and crush them to avoid choking. Watch out for any signs of an allergic reaction and seek urgent medical advice if necessary.

- **Salt** avoid adding salt to your child's food. Between the ages of one and three, a child's diet should contain no more than 2g per day. Ideally, you should restrict your salt intake too as it can contribute to high blood pressure. Processed foods are often high in salt – it is worth avoiding these where possible and keeping to the low-salt options for yourself and your child if you do use them.

- **Honey and sugar** avoid adding them to foods to make them more appetising. They provide empty calories and encourage a 'sweet tooth'. Also, honey should not be given under the age of one, as there is a very small risk of it causing the serious bowel infection botulism.

- **Sugary and fizzy drinks** can cause dental problems and again feed a sweet tooth. Go for no added sugar options and stick to water or milk between meals.

- **Skimmed milk** doesn't offer enough vitamin A or calories for the under fives. They can have semi-skimmed milk from the age of two as long as they are eating a well-balanced diet.

supplement. If you are carrying more than one baby, from the twelfth week onwards, you should be taking a daily supplement that provides 15 mg zinc, 2 mg copper, 250 mg calcium, 2 mg vitamin B_6, 300 mcg folic acid, 50 mg vitamin C, 5 mcg vitamin D and 30 mg iron.

Problematical foods and drink

You need a healthy balance of foods while pregnant, but there are some foods you should either eat with caution or avoid altogether.

Meat

Only eat meat that is thoroughly cooked (no tartare dishes or Parma ham) and has no trace of blood left in it – order "medium-well" to "well done". You need to be particularly careful with poultry. Avoid liver as it can contain large amounts of vitamin A, which can be harmful to the developing baby. This is particularly important if you are taking a vitamin supplement (as these contain more vitamin A).

Eggs

These should be cooked so that both the yolk and the white are solid, not runny, to avoid the risks of salmonella, which causes food poisoning. This rule applies for toddlers too.

Bear in mind that this means avoiding home-made mayonnaise, mousses, ice cream and other foods that may contain undercooked eggs. Shop-bought versions are usually safe to eat but be wary in restaurants.

Fish

Raw fish or sushi may contain tiny worms although most sushi sold in supermarkets is made with frozen fish, which is safe to eat. But if in doubt, don't eat. Smoked salmon is considered safe to eat in the UK.

High levels of naturally occurring mercury can be found in some fish – swordfish, tilefish, king mackerel, shark and marlin. Too much mercury can damage the baby's developing nervous system and so these fish should be avoided. Tuna should also be limited to four medium-sized cans (each 140g drained weight) or two fresh steaks per week.

Shellfish

Avoid all raw or undercooked seafood, which can cause food poisoning. This applies to young children too.

Cheese

There is a risk of listeria infection with some soft types of cheese – those made with unpasteurised milk. Avoid feta, mould-ripened cheeses such as Brie and Camembert, and blue-veined cheeses such as Stilton and Danish Blue (even if pasteurised).

Milk

Only have pasteurised milk. Do not drink sheep's or goat's milk and avoid foods that contain them or unpasteurised milk.

Peanuts

Current advice is that you can eat peanuts in pregnancy as long as you are not allergic to them. In the past, some experts advised that peanuts should be avoided if there was a family history of allergy, but research has shown that eating peanuts in pregnancy does not increase the risk of your baby developing a peanut allergy.

Pâté

All freshly made pâtés should be avoided – even fish and vegetable ones as they can contain listeria the bacteria that causes listeriosis, an illness that has serious side effects for a pregnant woman and her baby.

Ready-to-eat meals

Avoid any that can't be reheated safely; any that have been partly cooked or fully pre-prepared for reheating at home must be cooked through until piping hot to kill any harmful bacteria.

Caffeine

There is no need to cut out caffeine altogether, but it is recommended that you keep your intake to less than 200mg per day. The risks are small, but large amounts of caffeine are thought to be associated with low birth weight and may also increase the risk of miscarriage.

As a guide:

- One mug of instant coffee contains 100mg of caffeine; a mug of filter coffee has about 140mg;
- One mug of tea contains 75mg caffeine;
- One can of cola has 40mg;
- 50g plain chocolate has 50mg; 50g milk chocolate contains 25mg.

However, drinks prepared in coffee bars are usually of larger sizes and may contain more caffeine than the above.

Drink as much water as you can, but you can also cut down your caffeine intake replacing caffeine-rich drinks with decaffeinated coffee, tea and juice.

Many cold and flu medicines contain caffeine so it is worth checking the label and talking to your doctor or pharmacist if you have any concerns.

Alcohol

The ideal is to cut out alcohol altogether; otherwise limit yourself to no more than 1–2 units once or twice a week. The standard glass of wine served in pubs and restaurants contains about 2 units.

Food preparation

The usual safety rules apply. Fruit, vegetables and salad should be washed carefully as soil, even small amounts, can contain the organism that can cause toxoplasmosis, an infection potentially very damaging to a developing baby.

Wash your hands after handling raw meat and poultry and keep separate chopping boards for meats and other foods. As always, take care cleaning down surfaces where you have been preparing meat.

Store foods in the refrigerator at the right temperature, checking that your fridge is below 5°C (40°F). Make sure any raw meat or fish is wrapped or stored in containers away from foods on which they may drip and placed in the coldest part of the fridge along with other perishable foods.

Certain products used in the kitchen including plastic containers and wraps can contain bisphenol-

A (BPA), a synthetically produced hormonal substance which is added to plastics to make them stronger but can cause problems with a developing fetus and growing baby. This chemical can migrate into food and milk (hence the campaign to stop selling baby bottles made with it) if the material is scratched or worn. Other plastic materials, such as polyvinyl chloride (PVC) and polystyrene may also be dangerous to you and your developing baby.

You should therefore not reuse any plastic packaging nor wash, boil or clean any plastic containers in the dishwasher unless they are marked dishwasher safe. Do not let cling film touch the food you are heating in a microwave.

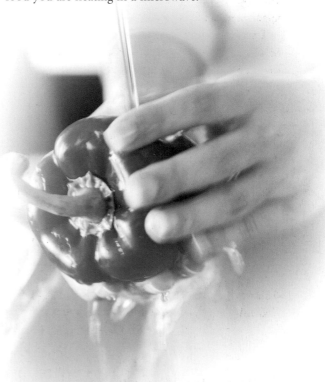

Your exercise routine

Exercise is an important part of a healthy pregnancy. It will boost your energy levels as well as helping to build up muscle tone and reduce constipation. It helps ensure that your muscles provide support for your growing baby and that they are able to expel her easily at the time of delivery. Being fit before the birth will help you also to get back in shape much more quickly afterwards.

Try to fit in 30 minutes of exercise 3-4 times a week and every day if possible. This could be as simple as taking a walk. If you are already fit, continue your fitness routine as long as you feel comfortable doing it. This is not the time to take up a strenuous form of exercise for the first time. If you are starting a new regime with your doctor's blessing, wait until the second trimester, when the risk of miscarriage is less. You should talk to your doctor or midwife if you have any concerns. If you go to classes make sure your teacher knows you are pregnant. Don't exercise to lose weight at this time.

Choosing your exercise

Low-impact exercise such as a stationary bike, yoga and swimming are ideal for pregnant women. They build up stamina and strength without putting strain on your joints. Anything that puts you at a higher risk of falling on or hitting your belly (like downhill skiing) is best avoided. High-impact aerobics will put too much of a strain on your joints at this time. If you are used to exercising with weights, change to machines as there is less of a chance that a weight can fall on your belly.

If you are expecting twins, walking and swimming will be your best options. Towards the end of your pregnancy, you'll probably find that walking is the most you'll be able to manage.
If you can afford it, it is a good idea to join a fitness club that offers classes and a crèche, so that your little one is looked after while you exercise. Alternatively, some centres offer mum and baby classes; swimming, yoga and pilates can usually be done together.

8 tips for exercising

1 Remember, with all forms of exercise, to ensure that teachers and coaches are fully qualified and that they know you are pregnant. They will be able to advise you what is appropriate for you at each stage of your pregnancy. Look for classes run specifically for pregnant women.

2 Wear comfortable clothing that is loose and doesn't restrict your movements.

3 Drink plenty of water and avoid getting too hot – overheating is not good for the developing fetus, particularly in the first trimester. Do not exercise in hot, humid conditions.

4 Take care of your joints. You may be more at risk of joint and ligament injuries as joints tend to be looser in pregnancy.

5 Avoid contact sports and those where you may fall and hurt yourself.

6 Avoid lying completely flat on your back. This may make you feel dizzy.

7 Remember tiredness is common in pregnancy so don't overdo things. Listen to what your body tells you.

8 Always warm up and cool down appropriately.

Yoga

This is great for your muscles and is a low impact exercise (doesn't put too much pressure on the joints). Yoga will make you more flexible and help your posture. These benefits combined with the breathing exercises you will do should help you cope better both mentally and physically with your labour. Once you've learned some basic techniques, you will be able to practice yoga while your child plays beside you on the floor.

Walking

Aim for a brisk walk of about 2 km three times a week. You will feel invigorated by the fresh air and the exercise – you may even find a brisk walk outdoors helps relieve morning sickness. Make sure, however, to pay attention to your posture and to wear comfortable shoes.

Walking is an easy way to exercise with your child; you can make it more interesting for her if you turn it into a learning experience – pointing out and collecting things from nature, for example.

Swimming

Often viewed as the ideal exercise for the pregnant woman, swimming works the muscles while supporting your body – and your bump. It benefits the circulation and is a great way to relax. Antenatal classes are available at many pools. Aim to swim for 30 minutes, taking rests whenever you need them, three times a week. Spending time with your child in the water can also be a great way to relax.

You can swim throughout your pregnancy without putting your joints under strain.

Pilates

A form of exercise that combines flexibility and strength training, its slow, controlled exercises work on your body's core stabilising muscles and increase their flexibility. Because some of the exercises are not

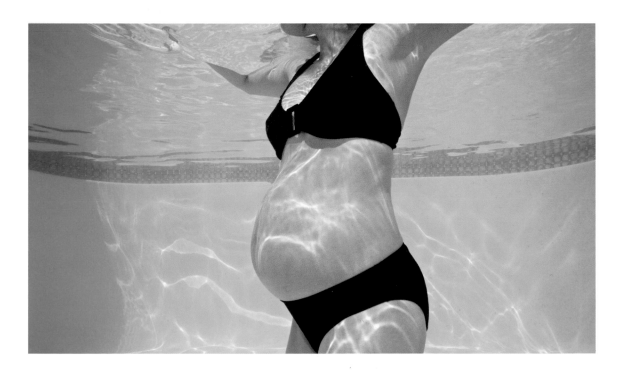

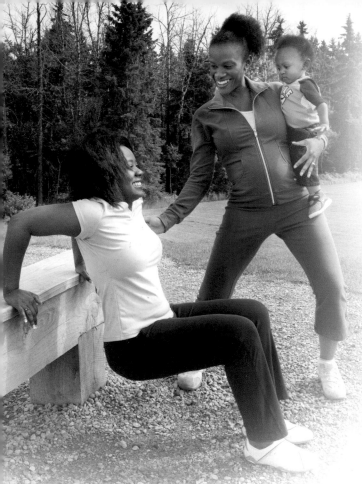

warming up and cooling down thoroughly. As you progress through pregnancy, you may be advised to cut down your running and possibly to walk in the last few months. It is worth listening to expert advice – and to your body.

Safeguarding perineal musculature

The pelvic floor muscles run from the pubic bone at the front to the bottom of your spine at the back (see page 24). They support the bladder and urethra and control the flow of urine; you use them when you squeeze to stop the flow of urine. Weakness of the pelvic floor muscles, therefore, can result in leakage of urine when the pressure on the bladder is increased, which happens when you laugh, cough or sneeze and jump up and down.

The pelvic floor muscles become weaker with every pregnancy and maintaining good urine control can take quite a bit of work. Moreover, increasing age hastens the deterioration of the perineal muscles. If you are expecting twins, the pelvic floor is subject to additional strain. For all these reasons, it more important than ever that you take steps to look after the perineal muscles and keep them toned.

Looking after your pelvic floor

It is very simple to strengthen these muscles. Just sit comfortably with your knees slightly apart and try to draw up the muscles, as if you were sucking something in. Hold for a few seconds, then release. Repeat at least 10 times. Do this several times a day, gradually building up the number of sets of exercises you do and holding each squeeze for longer. You can also exercise the muscles when standing and lying down (see page 97) – and since no one can tell when you are doing this – you can perform the exercise at your desk, when riding in a lift or on an escalator or even when chatting on the phone.

Focus on squeezing the correct muscles and keeping the stomach and buttock muscles relaxed. Keep breathing as normal. Once you are used to doing the exercises they will become a routine part of your day and you will be able to work on your pelvic floor during most of your normal activities.

suitable from mid-pregnancy onwards, you should be supervised to ensure you are performing safely. Pilates is also a great way of getting back in shape post-pregnancy. There are mat versions of the exercises, which once mastered, can be repeated safely at home while your child can play alongside.

Running

If you ran regularly before you became pregnant, continuing to run will be a great way to work your cardiovascular system. However, running is a high-impact exercise and pregnancy is not the time to start. Brisk walking is a great and less strenuous alternative to give yourself a cardio workout and you can build up gradually.

Running or walking with a buggy means that you can take exercise while spending valuable time with your child. Try to run or walk on flat ground as the change in your balance when you have a bump may make you trip more easily. Protect your muscles by

Relaxation

Being able to rest body and mind may be even more important in a second pregnancy than a first – though harder to achieve. While you have the maturity and experience not to be stressed by many of the worries and fears you had first time around, you have the extra responsibility of caring for a young child, which can take up the majority of your day. You need to seize your chances for sitting with your feet up.

If your child is young and still naps during the day, try to take advantage of his down time by resting yourself rather than catching up with chores. If you do have cooking or cleaning to do, wait until he's awake and get him to help you – giving him a dustpan and brush can keep him occupied while you're in the kitchen, for example.

Put aside some of the day for a quiet reading or story time session. Get cosy in a chair or bed and relax while reading aloud or telling stories. Or, you can listen together to an audio tape or some music. If you have a baby or older toddler who enjoys baby massage, a session may be relaxing for you both and, if you're lucky, your child may even drop off to sleep at the end.

Having a bath provides a great chance to rest and relax – and the opportunity to spend time with your first child. Using a moisturising bath wash can combat the drying effects of the water.

In the evening, when your child's asleep, either have an early night or ask you partner to give you a back or foot massage, which can be very relaxing. If your child wakes during the night, make sure your partner attends to him.

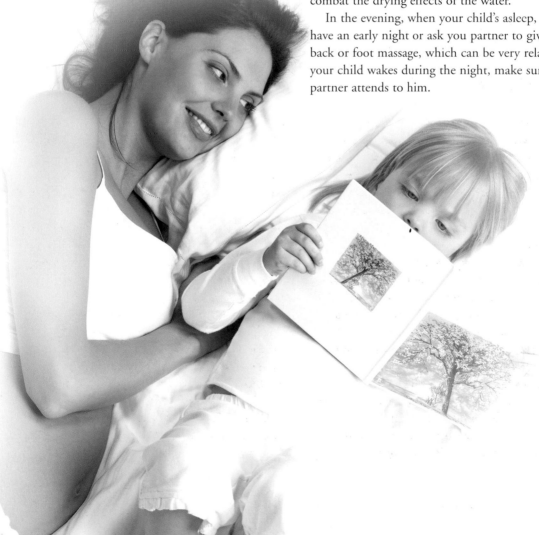

Lifting and carrying

Although the best advice might be not to lift or carry, particularly weights of 10 kilos (22 lbs) or more, it is almost impossible to avoid doing so, at least occasionally, particularly if you have a child. Bear in mind that you should never attempt to lift anything that will require you to strain. This is not because it would harm your baby, but to assure your continued comfort during the pregnancy. A strained muscle is never pleasant, but is especially undesirable during pregnancy. If at all possible, ask your partner or a friend to do any lifting or carrying, particularly once you are in your last trimester.

During pregnancy, changes to your body mean that your centre of gravity and muscle and joint fitness alter. The increase in body weight and the relaxation of your muscles and ligaments in preparation for baby's birth can make you off balance, which can lead to injury when lifting and carrying – even small items such as shopping bags.

Your back isn't the only thing that you have to consider. When you lift heavy things, you have a tendency to do something called a *val salva*. This is a manoeuvre that you make when you are really constipated and trying to have a bowel movement

FROM A STANDING POSITION

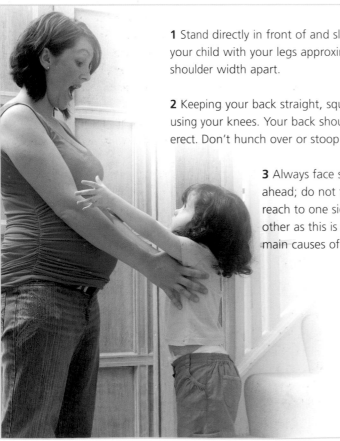

1 Stand directly in front of and slightly over your child with your legs approximately shoulder width apart.

2 Keeping your back straight, squat down using your knees. Your back should remain erect. Don't hunch over or stoop in any way.

3 Always face squarely ahead; do not twist or reach to one side or the other as this is one of the main causes of strains.

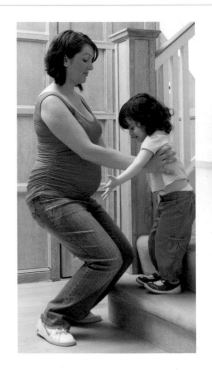

or when you are making a grunting sound. If you had a vaginal delivery with your first pregnancy, you made val salva movements while you were pushing your baby out (bearing down). These movements are usually of no consequence to your pregnancy, but there are a few situations where excessive val salva movements can potentially lead to problems. If you had something with your first pregnancy called an incompetent cervix (a condition where your cervix is too weak to hold the pregnancy), excessive val salva movements can increase the likelihood that this will happen again. Also, if your cervix is dilated because of preterm labor, doing these movements can cause the cervix to dilate more.

You can do some things to deal with these problems. First of all, just be mindful of these things when you have to lift something. Squat to pick something up rather than bending over. Second, while you are lifting or carrying something heavy, make sure you are breathing normally. It is impossible to val salva while you are breathing. And finally, as mentioned earlier in this chapter, regular exercise during pregnancy helps to build a strong back and lessens the chances of injury.

Certain women may even suffer from Symphysis Pubis Dysfunction (SPD), which is caused by the joints separating slightly due to the relaxing ligaments. If you've suffered with SPD before then you are more likely than average to develop it. If you do have SPD again, it may also appear earlier and worsen more quickly the next time around, so it's important that you see your doctor or midwife as soon as you have any symptoms.

Lifting

When picking up something from the floor or lifting your toddler, make sure you do so as you would for any heavy object, using your legs, not your back, to take the strain. If your child can manage it, and it is safe to do so, you might have him stand on a block or higher surface so you don't have to bend too far down.

You also will need to protect your back when placing your baby in and out of his car seat and cot.

Into and out of a car seat

If you have a two-door car, climb into the back seat next to the car seat with your baby held on your lap. Supporting him under his buttocks, lift him into his seat. Remove him by sitting next to his car seat, lifting him onto your lap and then leaving together.

Into and out of a cot

When putting him into or taking him out of his cot, generally the side rails will not lower sufficiently and you'll have to reach over the top to lay him down or pick him up. Take a wide stance and raise your back leg with your knee straight to maintain your spinal alignment.

4 Tuck your pelvis under as this adds strength to the lift. Try to clench your pelvic muscles (kegel exercise), as this strengthens your core and places the mechanics of the lifting into a stronger mode.

5 Pick up your child, and keep her close to your body. Support your child by holding her under her bottom.

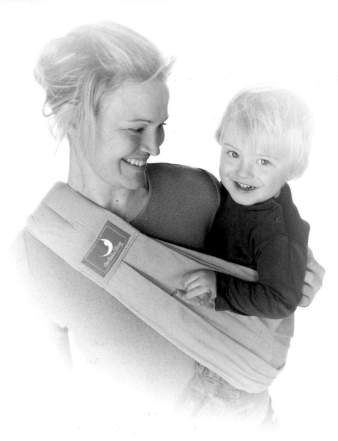

Carrying

Small children still want to be carried – and especially so when a new arrival is anticipated. Being held and carried close to you will reassure your youngster while still enabling you to do other things with your hands.

It is advisable to carry a baby on your back as soon as you can – but only once he has sufficient head control. If you carry your baby on your hip, make sure to switch hips regularly. The same is true if you normally carry your baby against one shoulder.

Many mothers find using a soft sling is the best solution as not only can you carry your toddler in a variety of ways – on your front, hip or back – but you can change the way you wrap it to accommodate your weight gain and changing shape. For example, it may be tied first above the belly and then, as your belly balloons, below. A soft wrap may make it easier to distribute your weight more evenly than a hard carrier would. Slings incorporating a ring are easy to tie in different ways and offer security against fabric slippage.

6 other occasions to squat or kneel

In addition to protecting your back when picking up your child, remember to bend down when

1 Picking up something from the floor.

2 Weeding, planting and doing other gardening chores.

3 Looking in the oven.

4 Opening lower cupboards and drawers.

5 Cleaning the floor or bathtub.

6 Washing your baby in the bathtub.

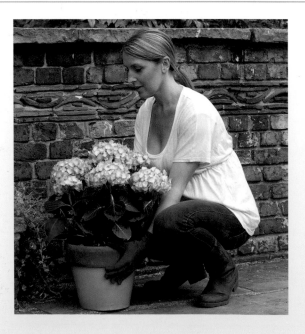

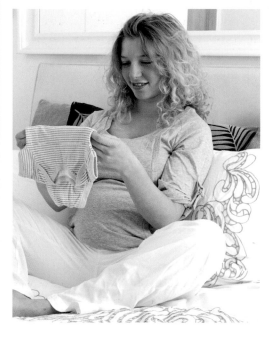

MAKE IT EASY ON YOUR BACK

- Don't bend over a bed to fold clothes. Instead, sit on the bed or move the items to a countertop.
- Remember to kneel when washing your child or take him in the tub with you – it's easier and more fun in the early months of pregnancy.
- Make sure the handle on your pushchair is at the proper height so that you are not bending over to propel it. When wheeling supermarket carts, keep the handle close to you, don't extend your arms.
- When performing tasks like vacuuming, mopping, sweeping or raking leaves, which involve using long-handled tools, work diagonally in the lunge position. If you are right-handed, put your left foot forward and extend your right arm (vice versa if you are left-handed). Keep your forward knee a little bent and push from your straightened back leg.
- When ironing, keep your feet apart and move back and forth between them or rest one foot on a low stool.

Taking care of your skin, hair and nails

Hormonal changes in pregnancy result in a number of changes to the skin, hair and nails. Generally, these are good: an increased blood supply to the face usually imparts a characteristic "glow"; decreased sebum production results in fewer spots and blemishes and some skin conditions such as eczema and psoriasis can improve. However, for some affected women, these latter two conditions can worsen and greater amounts of oestrogen in the bloodstream can result in increased body pigmentation (particularly for brunettes) and chloasma, in which facial skin darkens in patches, and

an increase in the number of moles and/or changes to existing ones. The hormonal changes can also make oily skin dry or dry skin oily so you may need to alter your normal skincare regime.

Most of the skin changes associated with pregnancy are no more or less common the second time around, but they may vary in intensity. The good news is that any stretch marks may be less noticeable than they were the first time since your skin, having been stretched from your previous pregnancy, is now a little more pliable. On the other hand, spider veins may be

6 simple tips to keep your skin in the best possible condition

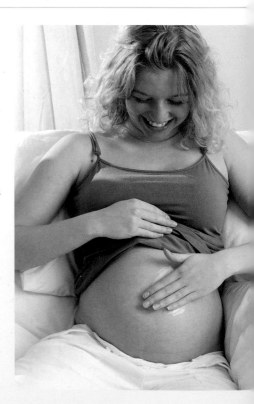

1 Make sure that your skin care products and make-up are suitable for use during pregnancy. Bone up on chemical terms and check the labels to ensure products don't contain harmful chemicals under other names. "Natural" is not a scientific term and can be misleading. If you're not sure, don't buy.

2 When choosing products look for the "Soil Association" logo, a sign that the product contains at least 95 per cent certified organic ingredients.

3 Use plenty of moisturiser, particularly on areas prone to dryness and stretch marks.

4 You may burn more easily so use higher factor sun creams and moisturisers and foundations that offer UV protection.

5 Soap can dry the skin and so should be replaced with a wash that moisturises.

6 Look after your feet with soaks and foot gels – tired feet are common in pregnancy and your feet deserve some special attention.

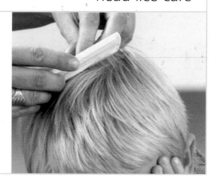

Though head lice are a bane of primary school children, do not use shampoos containing lindane (hexachlorocyclohexane) on yourself or your child. This organochlorine can build up in the uterus and ovaries and pass through the placenta and is extremely hazardous to health – both to you, your child and your developing baby. Ask your pharmacist for advice on what to use instead.

more noticeable because you have a greater propensity to develop these the older you are.

Hair may improve in texture or become thin and lank. Bear in mind that any treatments you apply to your air – colour and perms, for example – may produce a different result now.

Your nails can become brittle and rise from the nail bed. Massaging baby oil into your cuticles can help.

If you are in your thirties, expected skin changes may also be accompanied by the first real signs of ageing – fine, dry lines around the eyes and tiny red dots (broken veins) and "smile" lines running deeper on the side you sleep on. These changes are caused by decreasing collagen and elastin fibres and increased water loss. Stress may also be a factor. Pregnancy is not a good time to use anti-wrinkle creams that contain vitamin A (retinol) as an excess of this vitamin can cause birth defects.

Unwanted chemicals

Hardly a day goes by without news of an environmental toxin, which could be dangerous to your body or your baby. These occur not only in your food (see page 52), but also in cleaning products, some baby bottles and in cosmetics and skincare products.

The main culprits are phthalates, which are hormone disrupting but are easily absorbed through the skin. The most frequently used phthalate in cosmetics, DBP, is also the most potentially harmful, capable of affecting a baby boy's reproductive system. It is found in skin lotions, perfume, night creams, sunscreens, mascara and deodorants. Parabens, the most widely used synthetic preservatives, are found in skin creams, face masks, foundations and deodorants. Traces of these chemicals have been found in breast tissue, making it likely they can be transferred in breast milk.

SAFER SKIN AND HAIR CARE AND COSMETICS

The following brands produce products free from the 3 Ps – petrochemicals, parabens and phthalates – as well as artificial colourings, flavourings and other questionable additives.

Neal's Yard Remedies

Ren

The Organic Pharmacy

Green People

Spiezia Organics

Jurlique

Dr. Hauschka

Weleda

Aveda

Daniel Galvin Junior

Creating a relationship with your baby before birth

Creating a relationship with your second baby during pregnancy brings many benefits. Bonding is vital to infant development and the earlier it starts, the better. If the relationship begins before birth, the chances are that it will continue after your baby is born. You'll also have a more positive attitude to your second pregnancy once you feel there is a psychological connection between you and the baby in the womb. This may be particularly important if, for example, you are disappointed to have discovered that your second baby isn't the gender you had hoped for, or if this second pregnancy was unplanned and you had anticipated a larger age gap between your first and second child.

But forming an emotional connection, a psychological relationship, with your second baby while he's still in the womb is unlikely to happen instantly – even if it did with your first pregnancy. This type of attachment can take more time to develop with your second baby and the primary reason you probably won't feel the same this time round is because you are busy caring for your first child and have less time for yourself than you did when first pregnant. That's perfectly normal; you have to deal with the practicalities of everyday life, which, by necessity, means you have less time for your unborn baby. Furthermore, the novelty of the experience is not as vivid as it was previously.

While it is important to try and form a connection, don't feel pressurised into pretending to experience emotions that are, in fact, not there. Just relax and be yourself. Rest assured that the relationship between you and your baby will form gradually and steadily during the pregnancy, even if it feels different this time. Have confidence in yourself and your skills as a loving parent. It can also help if you engage in the bonding activities set out below.

Making the connection

In addition to your body providing nourishment and a safe environment in which your baby develops from conception to delivery, you also have a psychological connection. Your baby's senses are linked to your senses, and through them, his emotions are linked to your emotions.

Take hearing for example. Researchers using electrical recordings of brain waves have proved that a fetus can respond to sounds from as early as six months following conception – perhaps even a couple of months earlier. This means your baby's hearing is up and running at least three or four months before he will be born. Ultrasound images also reveal that, from the age of seven months onwards, when a fetus hears a sound, he will almost certainly close his eyelids in response – his way of showing that he is listening.

Another study involved a group of pregnant women, each of whom made a tape recording of herself reading three children's stories. The researcher then chose one of those stories and the mother played only that story on the tape recorder several times a day from the sixth month of her pregnancy onwards. As soon as her baby was delivered, the researcher then played all three previously recorded stories to the newborn. The results were astonishing – the baby was unresponsive to the two unfamiliar stories but began sucking vigorously as soon as he heard the story that had been read to him during the pregnancy.

It's not surprising, therefore, that many pregnant women find a clear connection between exterior noise and fetal activity. You may find that during your pregnancy your baby becomes more active while you listen to loud music or when you are at the movies. You might even feel your baby give a startled kick when you hear a very loud, sharp unexpected noise.

Of course, nobody is precisely sure what a baby hears while inside the womb. Sound does not travel well through fluid and therefore any sounds he picks up are likely to be very muffled. In addition, his outer ears are covered with a thin layer of vernix, which is a creamy protective substance. Even though sound inside the womb is probably quite unclear, hearing your soothing familiar voice while still in the womb will have a calming effect on your growing baby.

Similarly with hearing, tension, stress and anger will also be felt by your baby – from as young as four months – according to some scientists. Although this psychological link between you and your unborn baby is not direct, most professionals agree that the emotional wellbeing of the two of you is linked.

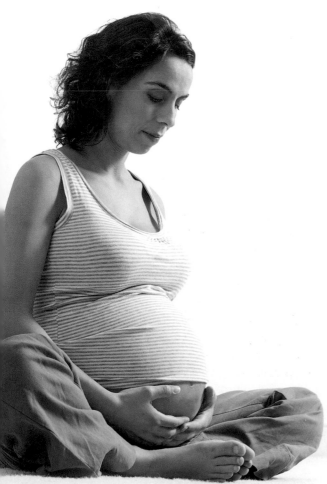

Start talking

The most effective way of creating a relationship with your baby in the womb is by talking to him. It really is as simple as that. Get into the habit of talking out loud to your growing baby during the day, either at work or while you are taking care of household tasks. Describe what you are doing, no matter how trivial the job might seem to you. Work on the assumption that while your baby can't hear every word clearly, and while he couldn't even understand the meaning of the words if he could hear them, he does hear something and he does feel the vibrations of sound. He is soothed, reassured and probably entertained by the sensations associated with your spoken words.

Consider reading stories to him as well. That may seem odd at first but you'll soon get used to it. When you have a few moments to relax and rest with your feet up, try to find some time to read a children's story out loud. Recite this as if you were reading it to a child who was in front of you, listening and following every word. Vary your tone of voice appropriately in line with the narrative. The more regularly you do this, the more your baby will get used to the experience – and familiarity usually has a comforting, calming effect.

Listen to music together

Make a point of playing your favourite music during your second pregnancy. Not only will this calm and relax you (assuming you choose something easy to listen to rather than heavy rock), it will also relax your baby. Shared emotional experiences such as this strengthen the emotional attachment between you and your unborn baby. Although your baby hears bass frequencies more clearly than other frequencies, there is no need to have the volume turned up or to place your "bump" right up against the sound source; if you can hear the music, your baby can, too. Be prepared to vary the music; blues, jazz, folk, operatic, classical, orchestral and contemporary will all be suitable. You may start to notice that your baby responds more to a particular type; babies have preferences too! And just as some studies revealed that new babies recognise stories they hear in utero, other research has found a similar effect with music – in fact, there is evidence that music heard in the womb is remembered up to a year later.

There is, however, no evidence that playing music to your baby in utero will make him more intelligent, despite the many claims that have been made about this. And if you play music during your pregnancy for the sole purpose of making your baby smarter, you will set yourself up for false expectations, which, in turn, may damage your relationship with him. Instead, listen to music for fun, and for the pleasure of knowing that you and your baby are sharing this pleasurable activity together.

Respond to physical activity

A baby in the womb typically starts to make his first kick around four months after conception, give or take a few weeks. One of the advantages of being a second-time-around mum is that you are more likely to recognise these early physical movements for what they are – first-time mothers often dismiss them as tummy rumblings, hunger pangs or indigestion. Aside from your baby testing out his newly developing skills, kicking is another potential form of communication with you.

Show your baby that you feel his kicks – perhaps by moving your position slightly or maybe even by gently tapping your tummy the same number of times that he kicks. Whatever you do in response – even if you speak out loud to him – your reaction helps form a connection with him while he is still in the womb. These touch activities are good fun for you, and hopefully for your baby, too. Some mothers are convinced that if they tap in a particular place, that's exactly where their baby will kick back.

Bear in mind that your fetus sleeps for around 90 per cent of the time, although that reduces slightly as the birth draws very near. While dozing, he is in a very deep sleep, often dreaming. Awake or sleeping, however, he might move up to 50 times an hour, so it's not surprising you feel something going on inside. Your awareness of his kicking and other movements depends on what you are doing at the time – you're more likely to notice them when you are resting quietly than when you are on the move.

You'll gradually get to know his kicking patterns and, as time passes, his kicks will become stronger and stronger.

During prenatal examinations, you'll have the opportunity to listen to your baby's heartbeat. The rate may be much faster than you expect (between 120 and 180 beats per minute – a bit like the sound of a horse in full gallop). Listen whenever you can as hearing the regular rhythmic beating sounds of your baby's heartbeat will make you feel even closer to him. The medical staff supervising you through your pregnancy may provide you with a mechanical device for listening to his heartbeat while you are at home – that's even better, as you don't have to wait for an appointment.

Give your baby an identity

Another way to strengthen the in-utero connection between you and you baby is by "making him real". The more your baby is an actual person to you, the closer you'll become with each other. That's why giving him a pre-birth nickname is helpful because it allows you talk about him in an affectionate, very personal way. (The nickname – for instance, Bump or Sweetpea – doesn't have to have any connection with the name you eventually give him once he is born.) This device is even more powerful when you and your partner use the nickname when in conversation with each other.

Keeping a diary of your baby's progress in the womb has a similar effect. Noting down key moments of each trimester, what is discussed at each clinic visit, what the different tests reveal, and so on, harnesses your interest, attention and enthusiasm. Years later, your baby will probably be delighted to read all those details about his development before he was born and he'll bask in the knowledge that you cared enough about him even then to keep a record of all that information.

5 TAKING CARE OF YOUR HOME AND OTHERS

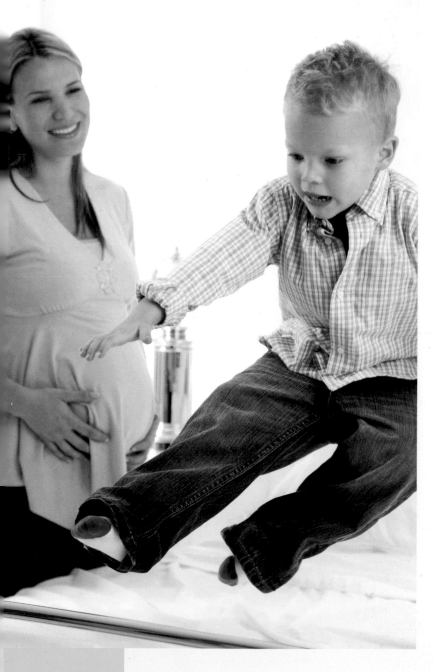

Being "super mum" is no longer regarded as a desirable or enviable occupation, particularly when you are pregnant. However, its important that your home is ready for the new arrival and that you follow recommended guidelines when looking after your older child, particularly if he becomes ill. You also should be taking steps to ensure your existing child knows about his expected new sibling. With all this going on, you may find it hard to maintain your relationship with your partner, but there are ways to ensure you face second parenthood as a couple.

Getting your home ready

As this is your second child, you will already know quite a bit about preparing for a new baby. Still, the arrival of your second baby (and possibly a third) will mean more changes, which will need to be thought through. You may need to move your first child to another room or, if she is staying put, to prepare a second nursery room.

You may be planning to have your new baby sleep in your room for a while, perhaps until he is sleeping through the night. But it is still a good idea to prepare the nursery now so you are ready when the time comes for him to sleep on his own. It will also be convenient to have a separate room straight away for nappy changing and storing toys and clothes. You may also wish to put a comfortable chair in there so that you or your partner can relax in it later on.

If your first child is moving from the nursery to her own room, it is important to make the move

well before the birth of her new brother or sister. This will ensure she has settled in plenty of time before the new arrival and doesn't feel that the new baby is taking over her room. If she is old enough, it's a good idea to let her help choose the decor and furniture for her room.

Preparing the nursery

Getting your home ready for your new baby will be a really enjoyable task for you and your partner. If your first child is staying in her own room, you will have a new nursery to prepare but if it's your older child who is moving, you may have to update the existing

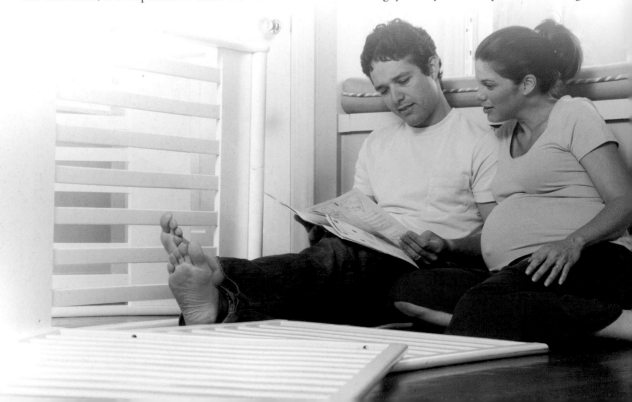

ASSEMBLING THE BASICS

Once your new baby comes home, you are going to have two (or more) children to take care of, so your time to get the shopping done will be sparse. Get as many of the things you will need as possible for your new baby ahead of time – like nappies and formula (if using) – so they will be waiting for you when you get home. It is also a good idea to stock your pantry well in advance since you won't have tons of time to shop for groceries. Be sure to include things that can be prepared quickly and with little effort.

On-line shopping may be really helpful, since you can do this right from home!

You will have many of the essentials already, but will need to double–up on some items. Here are the basics as a reminder.

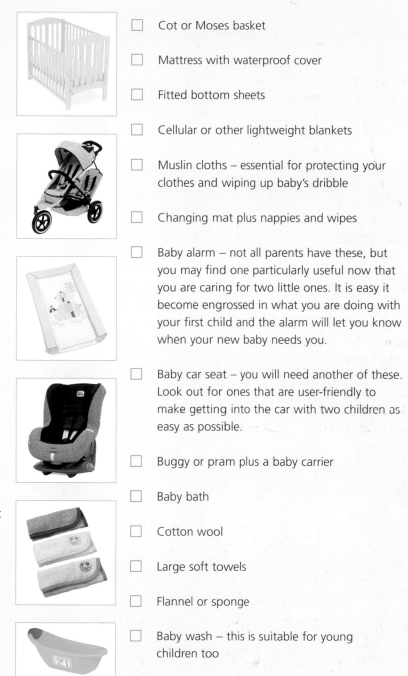

- ☐ Cot or Moses basket

- ☐ Mattress with waterproof cover

- ☐ Fitted bottom sheets

- ☐ Cellular or other lightweight blankets

- ☐ Muslin cloths – essential for protecting your clothes and wiping up baby's dribble

- ☐ Changing mat plus nappies and wipes

- ☐ Baby alarm – not all parents have these, but you may find one particularly useful now that you are caring for two little ones. It is easy it become engrossed in what you are doing with your first child and the alarm will let you know when your new baby needs you.

- ☐ Baby car seat – you will need another of these. Look out for ones that are user-friendly to make getting into the car with two children as easy as possible.

- ☐ Buggy or pram plus a baby carrier

- ☐ Baby bath

- ☐ Cotton wool

- ☐ Large soft towels

- ☐ Flannel or sponge

- ☐ Baby wash – this is suitable for young children too

- ☐ Baby hairbrush

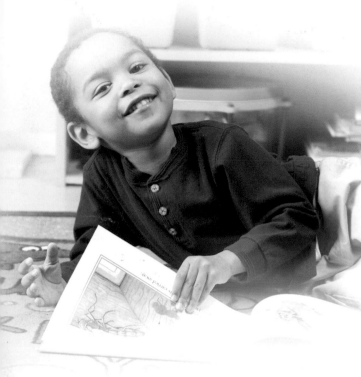

Whichever room is to be your child's for the whole of his childhood, it is a good idea to decorate it simply so that it can easily be updated as your child gets older.

Appraising your equipment needs

Having looked after one baby, you will have a good idea of what equipment works for you. This is the time to get rid of things you haven't found a use for and maybe invest in a few new items that could make your life easier.

You will also need to double-up on some items or buy additional equipment that caters for two children. For example, your single buggy will be fine for times you and your new baby go out alone. But, depending on the age of your first child, you may need a double buggy for when you all go out together. Many older children also enjoy riding on a step attached to the back of the buggy. Buying this and the double buggy plus using your original buggy will give you the flexibility to tailor your walks to your first child's mood and energy levels. A walk where your baby and child are able to drop off to sleep when they wish can be very relaxing for all of you.

You also need to consider whether you should buy a new cot mattress. Depending on the age of your existing cot, the mattress may not have a Kitemark tag proving that it meets current national safety standards.

You will also need an appropriate car seat to bring your newborn home. This should have a 5-point harness, be installed rearward facing in a seat not facing an airbag and be in place before you go to the hospital. If your baby (or babies) is pre-term, you'll need a first-stage infant car seat or a special padded insert that can support your baby in the seat.

One item you might like to do away with is a baby walker. According to *The Lancet*, they are of "no benefit to the baby", can cause accidents and may retard a baby's development.

If you are planning to bottlefeed you will need bottles, made of glass or non BPA plastic, teats, a steriliser, a bottle brush and maybe a bottle warmer. If you have existing plastic bottles but don't know if

nursery room and buy all new things for your first child. If, however, you only have one bedroom for your children, you will have to redecorate in order to accommodate the new arrival.

To make things easier for your first child, particularly if she is about to change from a cot to a bed, leave both items in his room. Although it may mean you have to use a cradle or Moses basket for the new arrival, your older child will have less of an adjustment to make.

If both children will be sharing a room, don't divide the room right away; by the time your new baby is ready to move out of your bedroom, your older child may be more interested in sharing. Once you do move the baby in, make sure there's a separate area and furniture to house your older child's toys and clothes.

Storage will be at a premium with two children and this is worth bearing in mind when you are choosing new furniture. If you're buying a bed for your older child, think about investing in bunk beds or a trundle bed, which your younger child can use later on.

they contain BPA, then it is best to throw them away. If you are going to breastfeed you will still need this equipment for the times you express milk, but you will also need a breast pump and pads.

Remember to think about how practical new equipment will be – for example, is the buggy easily collapsible, how light is it and how easy will it be to put into the boot of your car?

It is fine to buy some equipment second hand, but certain items like car seats and mattresses need to be bought new to ensure they are safe.

When buying clothes, limit the number of newborn baby grows, etc. you buy as most babies are this size for a very short time.

Making things safe

Even though you once made your home as child safe as possible, your first child may be sufficiently old enough that you felt certain protective actions were no longer necessary. Even if your existing child is a toddler, it's worth making another assessment before your new baby arrives to ensure you've thought of everything.

- Look carefully around your home with a toddler's eye view to identify any potential hazards.
- Make sure there are no sharp edges. Use corner cushions or foam on sharp corners.
- Think about fitting bars on any low windows and keep furniture that may act as steps for you child to climb up, like chairs, away from windows.
- Remove all mobiles, bumpers, pillows and duvets from the cot you will use.
- Make sure there are no trailing cords from blinds and shades that your baby can grasp by his bed or changing table.
- Make sure all rugs are non-slip.
- Plug plastic inserts into electrical sockets that are not in use.
- Hide long wires behind furniture.
- Leave electrical appliances unplugged so that your child cannot turn something on and hurt himself.
- Check existing smoke alarms for battery life and if you don't have any alarms, install some.
- Put safety locks on any cupboards containing potential hazards and on exterior doors.

FAMILY PETS

If you have a pet cat or dog it's worth taking some precautions. Even though your pet may be very fond of your first child, it may become jealous when a new baby joins the family and this may affect its behaviour. It's not uncommon for a house-trained animal to start having "accidents". It is a good idea to give your pet some special attention. However, you should keep all pets out of your baby's bedroom, put a net over your baby's pram if he is sleeping in it out in the garden to prevent your cat or others jumping in, have your pet wormed and wash your hands thoroughly after touching cat litter.

- Keep medicines, cleaning products, razor blades, and any other dangerous items locked away.
- Be careful with houseplants – you will need to ensure they are not poisonous and that they are not positioned where your child will easily be able to pull them on top of herself.
- Make sure any potential choking hazards, like coins and paper clips, are stored safely out of reach. Magnets are particularly dangerous when swallowed.
- Prop doors open or attach safety guards so little fingers do not get trapped.
- Don't put the TV on a table or chest, but make sure it is firmly fixed so your child cannot pull it on top of herself.

Breastfeeding while pregnant

It is possible to continue breastfeeding during pregnancy and it does give you the chance to sit and relax for a while with your first child. There have been concerns in the past about the possibility of breastfeeding triggering labour before a baby is due because of the action of oxytocin, but this is no longer thought to be the case.

Some women wean their existing child during the early part of pregnancy and then resume feeding once the new baby arrives. Others continue to breastfeed throughout pregnancy and then feed both their toddler and infant after the birth – known as tandem feeding. However, some women find breastfeeding and pregnancy too tiring to cope with and eventually decide to wean their older child.

If a child is to be weaned while you are pregnant, the most convenient time will be once he can drink from a cup and is on to solids.

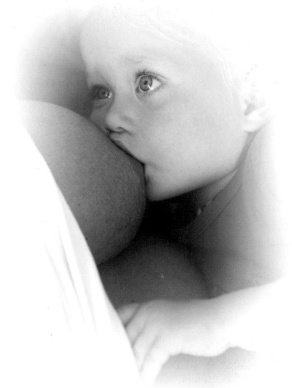

A changed experience

Even though you are already breastfeeding you may find that your nipples become sore again. Tender and swollen breasts normally occur during pregnancy. If you are breastfeeding at the time of conception, normal breast changes will manifest as a sudden increased sensitivity of the nipple. The nipple becomes extra sore and irritated while nursing, triggering pain and discomfort for many. Sometimes, this soreness is accompanied by feelings of restlessness and agitation. While the only cure for sore nipples is weaning, if you want to continue nursing, the soreness will gradually lessen as your pregnancy progresses.

Some women find that breastfeeding while pregnant can trigger nausea which is over and above regular morning sickness, particularly during the let-down.

Often a change to breastfeeding practices, such as experimenting with different positions, can help to overcome this.

There will also be changes in the quantity and quality of your breast milk. Pregnancy hormones cause a decreased milk supply – which is apparent

---

MORE **ABOUT** | oxytocin

This hormone that is released in response to a baby suckling and is responsible for the release of milk. It is also the hormone that sets off the contractions of the uterus when you go into labour. However, only very small amounts of oxytocin are released when breastfeeding and much larger amounts are needed to trigger contractions of the uterus. Also, experts believe that the womb only starts to respond to oxytocin after the 24th week of pregnancy.

from two to eight weeks after conception and continues throughout pregnancy until birth.

If you are breastfeeding an older baby who is on solids, the drop will be particularly noticeable but because the child can be weaned, it presents less of a problem than if your baby is under six months old.

If you have a young infant, you must take extra care to ensure he receives adequate nourishment. If your milk supply is too low, you may need supplementary formula. Discuss this with your healthcare provider.

The taste of your milk may also change and because of this, some children start taking less milk and gradually wean themselves at this time.

Being pregnant means that comfortable breastfeeding can be harder to achieve. Sore nipples are the first challenge and later your enlarged abdomen may make it difficult to find a comfortable position. Even given these potential discomforts, if you are determined and otherwise healthy, there's no reason why you can't continue to breastfeed.

Extra needs

If you breastfeed while pregnant, you need to take particularly good care of your body. As your body is supporting two growing babies, it requires extra rest and relaxation. Your diet is especially important as adequate nutrition and calorie content is crucial to cater for the needs of your first child, the developing baby and your own body (see also page 49).

You'll need to work closely with your caregiver when breastfeeding while pregnant. If you are anaemic, vegan, taking supplementary iron or having problems gaining weight, you may need supplemental nutrition.

For some situations, such as twin pregnancy or a history of premature labour, many doctors recommend weaning. In a normal pregnancy, extra care taken while breastfeeding results in healthy babies. Breastfeeding during a high-risk pregnancy, however, may involve risks for the fetus, which might outweigh the benefits for your breastfeeding child. If you are at increased risk of premature labour, your doctor will likely recommend that you wean your older child.

Weaning before birth

As mentioned previously, many children spontaneously wean themselves during pregnancy due to the changes in the taste of breast milk. Following the birth of your second baby, your milk will change further to suit the newborn. Your first child may want to stop breastfeeding at this time.

Like many mums, you may worry about weaning your older child and how he will cope with the loss of this special intimacy. Though there will probably be tears initially, with a positive approach and distractions, most children cope very well. It is important that you still spend time cuddling and being close so that the special times together continue. Discuss with your older child what he can do to help you and the new baby: he can talk and sing to baby, get nappies and wipes and get your water bottle. You can also use your breastfeeding sessions as storytelling times.

Tandem feeding

Some children, however, want the reassurance that being breastfed gives them and will want to continue. Feeding both your children at once can be difficult, but it is not impossible. Your milk supply will be adequate, but many women find the experience stressful. You will, however, need to experiment with finding a comfortable position. You can support your infant on a pillow and have your toddler sit, kneel or lie next to you.

At least initially, you should feed your newborn first as it is important she receives all the benefits of colostrum. Once your milk comes in, anything goes! You may decide to feed your children together or one after the other or a mixture of both.

Interestingly, engorgement is less of a problem this time around as you will have two children to empty the breast. If your toddler suckles first, it can be easier for your newborn to latch on.

Sometimes an older child who has been weaned or never been breastfed wants to have a go at the breast. Some women try to distract their child with a book or toy, others may express milk into a cup so their toddler can taste what its like or let the child suckle. The interest is usually short-lived.

Preparing your child for the new sibling

You should tell your first born child in advance that he's going to have a new brother or sister – don't wait until the last moment when labour has started, but don't tell him about the new baby when you are only a few weeks into your pregnancy. A child's sense of time is different from that of an adult; he may see no difference between a week and a month, or between one month and six months. And he may become bored with the long wait!

Start introducing the idea of the new baby when your abdomen is so large that even an inexperienced toddler would notice it, perhaps around the fifth or

6 ways to involve your child

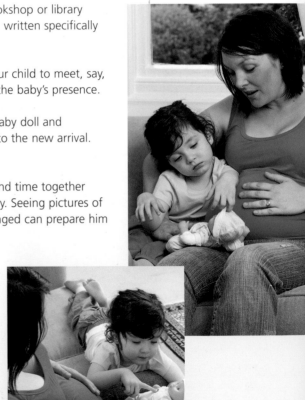

1   **Read him books about new babies** Your local bookshop or library should have a good selection of books on this topic, written specifically for young children.

2   **Get him used to new babies** Try to arrange for your child to meet, say, your friend's new baby so that he is comfortable in the baby's presence.

3   **Let him play "we have a new baby"** Buy him a baby doll and encourage him to pretend play being a big brother to the new arrival. Girls can practice being a big sister.

4   **Show him his "baby book" or family album** Spend time together looking at pictures of your child when he was a baby. Seeing pictures of him crying, being bathed or having his nappies changed can prepare him for what will happen when his new sibling arrives.

5   **Involve him in choosing the baby's name** You decide on the name, but present it to your older child in a way that makes him think he has made the choice with you.

6   **Let him help select baby items** If you need to buy new clothes, toys or equipment, take your child with you and ask him to help you select the things. Make it easy by narrowing the choice – which of two outfits, for example.

sixth month. Tell your child calmly, without feeling embarrassed about it. Pitch the conversation at a level suitable for his age and understanding, and avoid giving too many bits of information to him at the one time. For instance, it's better to say to him "I've got a terrific surprise for you. We're going to have a new baby soon" than to say, "I'm pregnant and in three months time I will have a baby". From the moment you first mention to your child that a new baby is on the way, use positive terms. Tell him the new baby loves him already and thinks he is a terrific older brother.

You might find that your child reacts with total indifference. Or he may seem very interested and want to talk about it further. Or he may simply burst into tears. Be prepared to let him ask you questions, either at the time you tell him or later — and always give him an honest, sensitive reply which will provide him with information and reassurance. For instance, if he asks "Where will baby sleep?", it's better to say "You will still have your bed, so we will get her a cot" than to say "We'll find somewhere, don't worry". Those early pre-delivery discussions and information-sharing sessions start to build your older child's involvement with your second baby.

If your child is still being breastfed and you expect to tandem feed (see pages 106-7), talk to your child about how he and the new baby will both be at the breast after the baby is born. Point out that since baby can't eat other foods like your toddler can, she will need to be fed more often. Show your toddler pictures of tandem feeding siblings.

If, however, your child has been weaned or you plan on breastfeeding your new baby and hadn't done so with your elder child, make opportunities for your toddler to see babies being breastfed. Explain that you will make milk for the baby, that breastfeeding is how a baby eats, and that it also helps a baby feel that she is loved and protected.

It's common for children to be curious about breastfeeding and it is not something you should hide from your older child. By seeing you feed, he is learning that breastfeeding is the normal, healthy way to feed a child rather than something that needs to be hidden.

Involving others

It may also be a good idea for your child to spend more time with your partner and/or other relatives and friends. Generally speaking, fathers spend more time on parenting and household chores once a second baby arrives, but you don't have to wait until he or she arrives to encourage your partner's participation.

It also makes sense to have grandparents on hand more too. The more used your older child is to being looked after by others, the better it will be for you once the new baby arrives. And, if you are planning to have a nanny or au pair, make sure he or she is familiar to your child before the new sibling arrives.

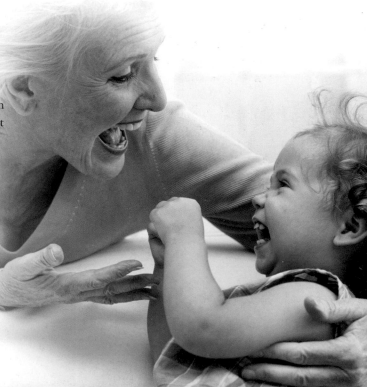

Looking after a sick child

Taking care of a child who is ill is worrying and time consuming at the best of times but if you are pregnant, you have the extra worry of wondering whether there is any risk of danger to your unborn baby. During pregnancy, a woman's immune system is naturally suppressed, which means that you are more likely to fall prey to infectious illnesses, and if you do so, you are more likely to develop complications including pneumonia (an infection of the lungs), difficulty breathing, and dehydration, particularly if you are in your second or third trimester. In rare cases, these problems can affect your unborn baby.

Most childhood illnesses, while distressing to you and your child, are not infectious. These include skin conditions such as allergic rashes and eczema, and bacterial infections such as impetigo. Most women, too, have been vaccinated against or have immunity to the childhood diseases – measles, rubella and chickenpox – that are most dangerous to a developing fetus. (Although contact your caregiver immediately if you suspect your child has any of these illnesses.) But flu, particularly swine flu, seems to put pregnant women at a higher risk for premature delivery, stillbirth and spontaneous abortion. The risks to the fetus are as yet unknown.

Flu, like other infectious diseases, is accompanied by fever. Studies have shown that a fever during the first trimester doubles the risk of neural tube defects in a fetus and may be associated with other adverse outcomes; anti-fever medications can reduce the risk of birth defects.

General precautions

Cold viruses are primarily spread from person to person in respiratory droplets of coughs and sneezes but they can also be picked up from inanimate objects – doorknobs, tissues, towels, etc. When caring for an ill child, therefore, it is important always to:

- Encourage your child to cover his nose and mouth when he coughs and sneezes. You should have plenty of tissues close at hand.
- Clean your hands with soap and water or an alcohol-based hand rub often and especially after handling any used tissues.
- Clean hard surfaces, such as door handles, toys and equipment, frequently using a normal cleaning product.
- Provide your child with his own towel and face cloths and keep these isolated from the others used by the rest of the family.
- Be prepared to keep your child somewhat isolated if he is suffering from a contagious illness. The ideal "sick" room should be free of clutter and be lit well so you can easily spot signs of worsening health.

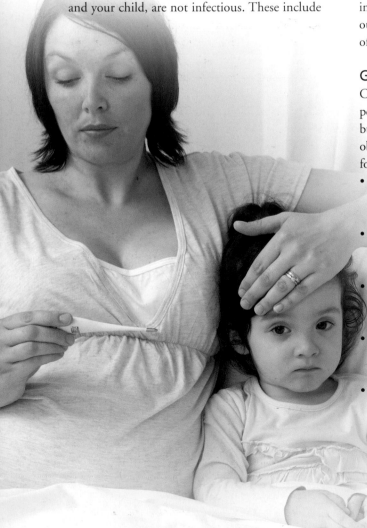

- Check with your health care provider about any special precautions you might need to take.
- Wear a facemask when you are close to your child.

Swine flu

As well as posing problems to pregnant women and possibly their unborn fetuses, swine flu is thought to put babies and toddlers at higher risk for severe illness. Therefore, it's important to recognize the symptoms. These include fever (a temperature of 38°C or above) and a cough, particularly if sudden onset, but also tiredness, headache, aching muscles, runny nose, sore throat, nausea and diarrhoea. If you suspect your child has swine flu, it is important to contact your doctor. He or she may prescribe antiviral medication (usually Relenza) as a prophylactic (preventative) measure. If possible, another well adult should care for your child. If you are diagnosed with swine flu, you will usually be given a course of the antiviral drug Relenza, which is inhaled using a disk-shaped inhaler. It is recommended for pregnant women because it easily reaches the throat and lungs, where it is needed, and does not reach significant levels in the blood or placenta. Relenza should not affect your pregnancy or your growing baby. However, if your doctor or midwife thinks that a different medicine is needed (for instance, if you have unusually severe flu), you may be given Tamiflu instead. An expert group reviewed the risk of antiviral treatment in pregnancy. It is much smaller than the risk posed by the symptoms of swine flu.

You can also take paracetamol-based cold remedies to reduce fever and other symptoms. Paracetamol is safe to take in pregnancy. However, you should not take non-steroidal anti-inflammatory drugs (NSAIDs) such as ibuprofen.

You should consider taking the swine flu vaccine as soon as it is offered. It will not harm you or your unborn baby.

Unless you have swine flu symptoms, carry on attending your antenatal appointments to monitor the progress of your pregnancy.

Digital thermometer

As fever can signal a condition dangerous to yourself and unborn baby, as well as to your child, you should have on hand a digital thermometer to take your child's temperature. This is placed in the mouth of toddlers and older children or in the armpit of babies.

HEALTH FIRST	german measles

Most children these days are vaccinated against rubella. If this is the case with your child, then you don't need to worry about him bringing it home. Most doctors test women at the beginning of pregnancy to see if they have been exposed to or vaccinated against rubella in the past by checking antibodies in the blood. If you have antibodies, then you can't get rubella and there is no risk to your developing baby. If you don't have antibodies, then your doctor will recommend that you get a vaccination to prevent problems in future pregnancies. Since you are reading this book, we are assuming that this is your second pregnancy and that if you did not have antibodies with your first, your doctor would have given you the vaccination, in which case there is nothing to worry about.

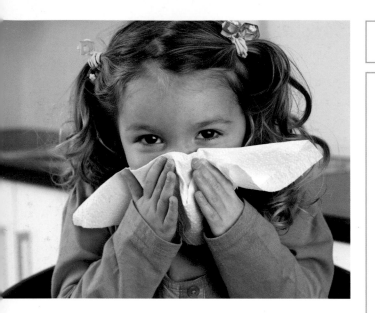

CYTOMEGALOVIRUS (CMV) INFECTION

This is an infection commonly suffered by children of preschool-age. The symptoms may mimic those of a cold or flu, like fever, chills and body aches, but many times there are no symptoms at all. By the time they reach reproductive age, about half of all women have antibodies to CMV in their blood, indicating that they have already had the infection even though they weren't aware of it. If you have had a CMV infection in the past, then the risk to your developing baby is extremely low. If, however, you get the infection for the first time while you are pregnant, the risk goes up. The risk is highest if you contract the infection in the first and early second trimesters of pregnancy because this is the period when the likelihood of passing the infection on to a fetus is greatest. Babies exposed during this time are at risk for developing hearing and visual problems, and sometimes even long-term learning difficulties. These problems are pretty rare, though, and only occur in 1/10,000-1/20,000 newborns.

Some doctors test for CMV antibodies at the beginning of pregnancy to see if women have been exposed in the past, especially if you are frequently around preschool children. If your child develops CMV or is exposed to someone who has it, you should limit direct contact with your child as much as is practically possible and be sure to wash your hands as often as possible. You should also let your doctor know, because if there is a chance that you have caught the infection during pregnancy, there are tests that can be done to see if the fetus has been infected – like amniocentesis and detailed ultrasounds.

Helpful environment

Small changes to your child's room can make it easier to care for him when he is ill. Try not to have him in your room or bed, if at all possible, but install a baby monitor, which not only can cut down on the number of times you need to check on him but can keep you touch. Place a supply of tissues, hand wipes and the thermometer in the room to save you having to go and get things frequently.

In the same vein, a coolbox containing water and/or juices will be handy in case you child has a fever. It could also be used to hold cooled-down water to use for sponging. Keep all medications, however, locked up in an inaccessible place.

Put up some brightly-coloured pictures that your child will enjoy, and make sure he has a supply of books and comics, and some simple toys that will keep him amused next to the bed. Audio tapes with stories and songs can be a help and you could bring in a tv and/or dvd player.

PARVOVIRUS INFECTION (FIFTH'S DISEASE)

This disorder is also common among preschool children. Flu-like symptoms such as fever, chills and a sore throat, followed by the appearance of a rash on the face that makes it look like the cheeks have been slapped, hence its other name, slapped cheek syndrome. Adults can also get the disease, the commonest symptoms being joint pain and stiffness, but some people have no symptoms at all. And, just like with CMV, most (over 75%) women have already been exposed to parvovirus in the past and have antibodies to it. If this is the case, then there is no risk to the developing baby. If, however, you haven't been exposed in the past and your little one develops it, let your doctor know because there is a risk that the fetus can get the infection, too. The main risk with a fetal parvovirus infection is transient anaemia. Most fetuses can tolerate this, but rarely, an

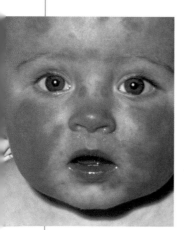

intrauterine transfusion is needed to treat severe anaemia. Your doctor will probably recommend that you undergo frequent ultrasound examinations to look for signs of fetal anaemia. The good news is that even if your baby needs a transfusion (and again, this is rare), the outcomes for these children are excellent.

CHICKEN POX (VARICELLA)

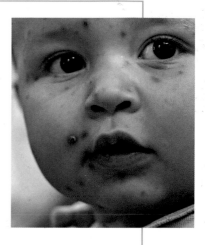

Chicken pox is highly contagious, so it is very likely that you already had the disease and have antibodies to it. Most children these days have been vaccinated against the disease, so the chances of being exposed are very low. If you don't have antibodies to varicella zoster (the virus that causes chicken pox), and you are exposed to it during pregnancy, let your doctor know as soon as possible so you can receive varicella zoster immune globulin (VZIG). This helps prevent transmitting the virus to your developing baby. It may also make your infection less severe, which is important since the symptoms in adults are often worse than they are in children. If you get the infection around the time of delivery, your baby's doctor may also give him VZIG to prevent the development of chicken pox in the newborn period.

Herpes zoster or shingles is also caused by the varicella virus. The lesions associated with this disorder contain some of the virus, so you should avoid contact if you are at risk for developing chicken pox.

Preserving your relationship with your partner

As a couple you will already have experienced overwhelming changes when you brought your first baby home. You will have had to cope with the stresses of becoming parents for the first time, including new responsibilities, changes in your everyday life, and a lack of sleep. Your new arrival may put new strains on your relationship with more demands being placed on you both and the return of broken sleep at night.

With all of this going on, it is no wonder that many new parents find their relationship suffers. It is important to spend time together, talking things through and showing each other that in all of this chaos, you still care for each other.

Make time to talk

The lack of sleep may make you irritable and this combined with having less time to spend together may have really challenged your relationship in the past. Hopefully you will have learned to make time for your partner and to take opportunities to spend time with each other with and without your child whenever possible. Communication is the key to maintaining a good relationship. It is very easy to be taken up with caring for your first child and now your pregnancy. If you are annoyed about something – and this applies to your partner too – make time to talk about it calmly rather than at a hectic time

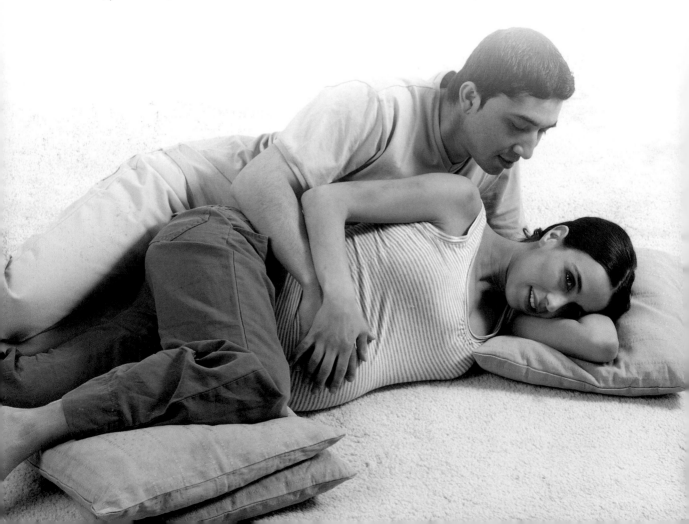

when your child is crying or needs you. Parents really need to work at finding time to focus on themselves as a couple. This will apply all the more when your second child is around.

Enjoy time as a family

You will also need time enjoying each other's company as a family. A leisurely walk with your baby in the buggy or time spent watching your toddler play in the sand pit at the park are opportunities to relax and chat.

Intimacy with your partner

It's likely that your sex life decreased after you had your first baby and this pregnancy is likely to diminish it even further. Even if you have a "normal" sex drive, fatigue, time constraints and possibly exhaustion from running around after a toddler, can get in the way of having sex. Some couples have intimacy problems when they have children or when the woman is pregnant. Some women feel less attractive when they are pregnant; others have problems thinking of themselves as a sexual being and see themselves only as a mother or a pregnant woman. Again, spending time together is the key to being close. It also enables you to have the reassurance from your partner that you are still loved and still attractive.

Try not to focus on whether or not you are having sex but try to enjoy time alone and think of gestures large or small that will help to keep romance in your relationship.

If, however, you or your partner are struggling with the lack of intimacy or if you have concerns about the effects sexual activity may have on your pregnancy, ask your healthcare provider. Don't be embarrassed to talk about your problems. Your doctor or midwife has dealt with these issues before and can offer advice to help address your concerns.

5 things to put you in the mood for sex

1 **Go to bed early.** While having an early night doesn't guarantee you'll feel like sex, particularly in the first minutes, you are more likely to become intimate if you go to before you're completely exhausted.

2 **Be creative.** You (or your partner) may not feel like sexual intercourse because of fatigue or other reasons, but there are many things that you can do to satisfy each other sexually besides intercourse.

3 **Make sure your child stays in his own bed.** Allowing a child in bed with you is a real put off when it comes to sex.

4 **Remove the TV from the bedroom.** Without this distraction, you may be able to better focus on your partner.

5 **Don't go to bed angry**. If you have problems with your partner, make sure you resolve them before going to bed. Otherwise, you won't be in the mood.

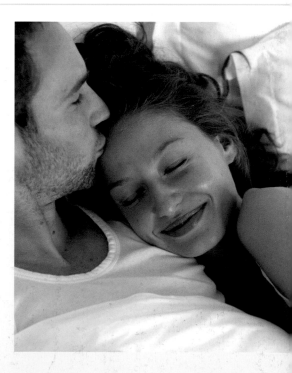

RELATIONSHIP AIDS

- Make time for each other – with your child and on your own as a couple.
- Accept offers from willing grandparents or close friends to watch over your child. Even just an hour or two together can make a big difference to how you feel.
- Share the workload, assigning particular tasks to one partner if that suits you, and praise yourself and each other for what you achieve.
- Be kind to yourself and each other – don't expect too much. You will both be tired at times. Give yourselves a break – don't worry if you leave the washing up overnight or don't dust your living room.
- Take care of each other – if your partner has had a bad day, small gestures like running him a bath and bathing your child when it's his turn could make a huge difference to how he feels. And he will do the same for you sometimes, too!
- Bear in mind you have immense hormonal changes going on in your body and with all that you are going through – low energy levels, morning sickness, back ache, change in sex drive, sore breasts to name but a few – it's no wonder that things seem to get on top of you sometimes. This is bound to affect your relationship at some time or another. Continue to spend time with your partner, relaxing and doing things you both enjoy. And try to be flexible as a couple. If you are feeling very tired or sick, rather than feeling annoyed and irritable with your partner resenting that you have to make his dinner, ask him to make his own dinner while you have a nap for an hour and then come back refreshed.
- And keep talking – your partner may have his own worries. This is a time for sharing and really supporting each other.

Sharing the care

Even if you have worked out how to share the care of your first child between you, now is an opportunity to revisit your schedules and talk through the way you do things to take account of your new baby's needs while still remembering your first child. If you were left with most of the responsibility the first time around, this is another opportunity to start sharing the care.

Much of how you will organise the care will probably evolve after your baby arrives and you all settle down together, but in the meantime you can start to make some plans, including how each of you will fit in spending time with your first child on her own so she gets opportunities to have your undivided attention.

Before your baby is born, it is a good idea to go out with your partner – to a restaurant or other neutral environment – to discuss what worked and didn't work the first time around. You could even make lists of various chores and situations.

Resolving issues

Always make time to iron out any issues. Letting things build up when you are tired and busy will only make for bigger problems later on. Be clear about what is bothering you and try to address conflicts as soon as possible.

If your child happens to catch you arguing, make sure she sees that you have made up so that she doesn't go off to bed feeling upset. Children should be aware that people can disagree and still love each other.

Caring for your relationship

As we have said, time together is the key. Ideally, schedule a time in your diary every week when you ask someone to care for your child while you go out together. Otherwise, cook each other a special meal once your child is in bed. You may have tried to start this routine with your first child but with busy lives it is all too easy to let plans slide. With your second child on the way, it is a good idea to try to reinstate this routine, making it a part of your normal life.

6 DELIVERY THE SECOND TIME AROUND

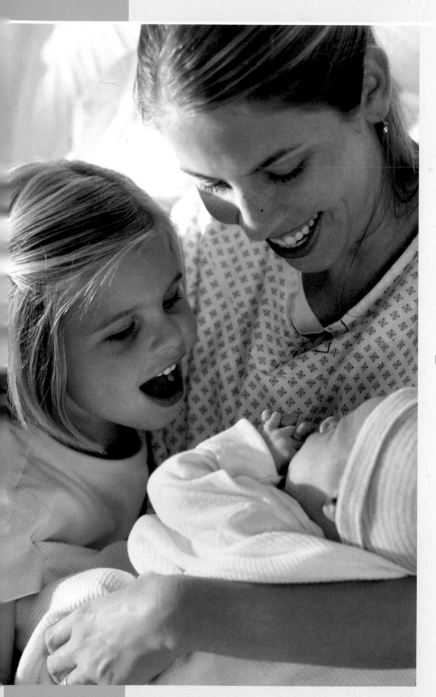

If you delivered vaginally the first time, the chances are very good that you will have another vaginal delivery. If you had a previous caesarean, you may be able to deliver vaginally this time or have a repeat procedure. What may be more within your control is where you choose to deliver your baby and whether you have your older child with you.

Choosing where and how to give birth

You may have had a wonderful experience with your last pregnancy and delivery and are planning on using the same hospital and/or midwife again. Many women who have had a midwife or consultant of their own choosing, feel a close bond to the person who delivered their child. However, even with a positive experience, you may find yourself needing to look for a new arrangement, or your previous experience may not have been what you expected, or the hospital may not have been what you imagined, and you are looking into other alternatives.

If you are working with an independent or private midwife, she'll assist you with your birth (in hospital or at home). Working with the same individual, (which is not usually available on the NHS) will enable you to build a trusting relationship, and to feel special and important. Knowing that the midwife who has provided you with antenatal care will be present at your baby's birth, and subsequently will care for you both following the birth, has a very positive impact on confidence levels. If a vaginal birth is planned, you will invariably deliver with less intervention and less pain relief. If you have seen your a consultant privately, he or she or a team midwife should be present at the birth.

If you choose or are advised to deliver your baby in hospital, you will be cared for by the labour ward team of midwives and then by the community midwives in the first few days following the birth. If

6 common reasons to seek a new arrangement

1 You moved and need someone closer to home or work.

2 You didn't have the experience you expected.

3 Your last pregnancy turned out to be complicated and now you need a high risk specialist, or your current pregnancy is considered high risk.

4 Your GP or midwife is no longer offering the care you need.

5 The hospital you delivered in before has closed.

6 You just didn't "click" with your last caregiver.

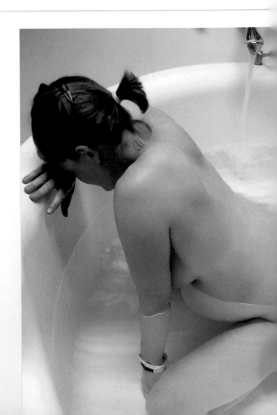

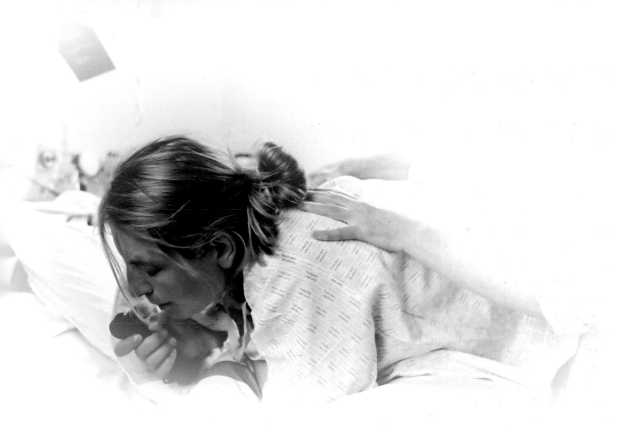

you are deemed 'suitable' to attend a midwife unit –
you are expecting your second baby after a problem-
free first vaginal birth – one of the team of midwives
will aim to deliver your baby. The team will also
look after you after the birth.

Hospital birth

Hospitals have made great strides in becoming more
welcoming and comfortable places in which to give
birth. However, they are still more likely to have a
conveyor-belt approach and to 'push' procedures
such as the use of oxytocin to progress labour. They
are also less likely than birthing centres to offer
water births. On the other hand, they are necessary
if special attention is required or if a caesarean is
planned.

Midwife unit birth

The care here is generally more personal since you
will probably have met at least some of the team.
The environment will be more homely, and there
will be less pressure for technical interventions.
Birthing pools are generally available. In the case of

a problem, if the unit is in a hospital, you will be
transferred to a different part where specialists can
look after you. If the unit it is located away from a
hospital, transportation to a nearby hospital will be
arranged. If the birthing centre is privately run,
there are often doctors are likely to be in attendance.

Home birth

While the vast majority of births occur within
hospitals, a small percentage of women choose to
undergo a home birth; in England, about 2.7 per
cent. Interestingly, women who have home births
are more likely to be older, and have had three or
more children already.

Some of these women may have had an
unplanned home birth, while others may have
specifically wished to avoid traditional antenatal care
and delivery in a hospital environment. If your first
child was born in hospital and you felt there was too
much medical intervention, you might be thinking
about having a different type of experience for your
second delivery, or perhaps you already had a home
birth and are considering this option again.

If you are thinking about a home birth, there are several issues to consider. First, your caregiver must advise that it is safe for you to deliver at home. With a second baby, this decision will be easier if you had a normal vaginal delivery the first time around. You would also need to find a healthcare professional who would be prepared to deliver you at home. Typically, home birth attendants are midwives but some GPs do home deliveries. As well as independent midwives, it is possible to be delivered by a midwife attached to the local hospital.

It is important to still receive antenatal care and testing. For a home birth, you should be at low risk for complications, have good support from a healthcare professional with appropriate experience, and also have a backup plan to ensure a smooth transfer to a hospital, if necessary. You should not consider a home birth if you are pregnant with twins, have underlying medical conditions (heart problems, kidney disease, diabetes, high blood pressure, etc.), are preterm, have obstetric complications (placenta praevia, bleeding,

pre-clampsia, etc.) or if the fetus is not in the vertex (head down) presentation.

Bear in mind that not all women attempting a home birth end up delivering at home. The most important thing to consider is your safety and the safety of your child. In one study carried out at London's Whittington Hospital about 10 per cent of women attempting home births needed to be transferred to the hospital before delivery. Some women are transferred for urgent reasons. Most studies suggest that planned home births involving low-risk women have reduced rates of caesarean section and medical interventions, with similar rates of perinatal morbidity and mortality compared to hospital births.

Baby's position

Most babies at term (96 per cent) are lying "head down" or in the vertex presentation. This is because under normal circumstances, the baby fits best in this position. The bulkiest parts of the body – the buttocks and legs – are in the roomiest part of the womb (the top or fundus). However, some babies are sitting in the breech presentation, meaning that their buttocks or feet are presenting closest to the cervix, while others are lying across in the uterus, in what is called "transverse lie". Breech and transverse lies are slightly more common in women who already have had a child, especially those who have had several children. One explanation for this is that the abdominal wall is more relaxed, and so the baby is not held as tightly or firmly in the head down position and can move about more freely.

If you had a breech baby the first time, the chance of another breech may again be higher if there is an anatomical explanation for your baby being breech. For example, if your uterus is an irregular shape (bicornuate [heart-shaped] or T-shaped), or if you have fibroids protruding into the uterine cavity, or if you have a long septum (dividing wall) within the uterus itself, the baby may not fit most comfortably in the head-down position, and since most of these problems will not change from one pregnancy to the next, a breech baby may be more likely to recur.

4 reasons for a home birth

1 Wanting to experience a low-intervention birth (avoiding induction of labour, anaesthesia or pain medicine and episiotomy).

2 A desire to deliver in the comfort of one's own home surrounded by family and friends.

3 Religious or cultural issues.

4 Greater privacy.

Non-recurring causes of a breech baby include increased amniotic fluid (polyhydramnios) or some fetal abnormalities. Because delivering a baby as a breech can be more complicated and associated with some higher short-term risks, many obstetricians will recommend either caesarean section or trying a procedure called an External Cephalic Version (ECV) to turn the baby to the vertex position. This involves manipulating the woman's abdomen and is performed at 37 to 38 weeks of pregnancy, when there is still sufficient amniotic fluid to allow for a small amount of movement.

ECV has over a 50 per cent success rate, and usually is easier to perform on women having their second or third babies, because the abdominal muscles are more relaxed. While there are some risks of performing ECV – for example, a drop in the fetal heart rate, detachment of the placenta from the wall of the uterus – these complications are unusual.

If ECV is not successful, or you choose not to try it, a caesarean section will be recommended as elective breech delivery is really uncommon.

Helping your baby to turn

If your baby is in a breech position or a transverse lie, it may be possible to help her to assume the head-down position by changing your position or using visualisation. No large-scale studies have been carried out but there is good anecdotal evidence to suggest that the following things can help.

Assuming postural inversion or a breech-tilt position, where your pelvis is higher than your stomach, for a minimum of 10 minutes twice a day can allow your baby's head to float, which will encourage her to turn so that her head moves up into the pelvis.

To assume the position, lie on your back with your knees flexed and place four plump pillows or cushions under your buttocks so that your pelvis is higher than your stomach. Alternatively, use the knee-chest position: kneel down on the floor with your buttocks raised as high as possible while your head rests on your folded arms.

Alternatively, some women have found it effective to simply imagine their babies turning. On an empty stomach, concentrate on relaxing your abdomen while visualising your baby turning. Repeat for 10 minutes twice a day.

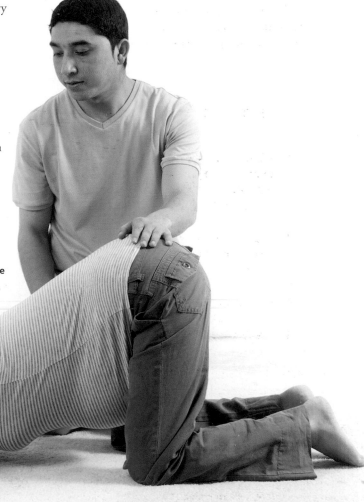

The knee-to-chest postion may help a breech baby to turn and creates space for him to get into a good position. The baby's bottom will move away from the mother's pubic bone and his spine becomes lower and flatter. Dr. Juliet DeSa Souza, retired professor of obstetrics and gynaecology at Grant Medical College, Bombay, found this method successful in a 1977 study.

Labour the second time around

The best (and worst) thing about delivering your second child is that you've been through it all before! Remembering the contractions, pain, pushing and recovery may make you cringe, but remembering the joy surrounding the arrival of your baby may flood your mind with beautiful memories. Most women feel less nervous and stressed about giving birth the second time. Knowing what to expect, whether or not you want pain medications and/or epidural anaesthesia and what the labour is all about is usually comforting. Bear in mind, though, that each labour is different. Fortunately, second labours are usually easier and faster than the first time around.

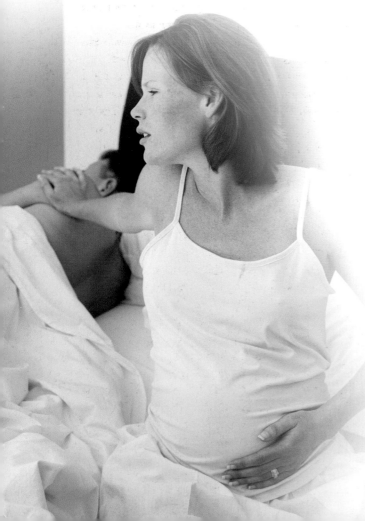

Recognising labour

In first pregnancies, women often do not dilate or efface (thin-out or shorten) their cervix until they go into labour. However, in a second pregnancy, you may walk around 2 to 3 cm dilated and almost fully effaced for weeks. Even though you experienced contractions before, you may not be sure whether you are truly in labour or not! Many women experience more frequent and stronger Braxton-Hicks contractions in their second pregnancy, and may be uncertain whether they are in actual labour. Don't worry or be embarrassed if you are unsure. It's always better to call your midwife and get checked out just in case.

Shorter first and second stage

The first stage of labour is from the onset of active labour to being fully dilated (10 cm) and the second stage is from full dilation to delivery (the stage when you are pushing). The good news is that both of these stages tend to be shorter the second time around.

The whole labour and delivery process usually takes about 12 to 14 hours for a first child, and about eight hours for the second. There are a few reasons for this. First, the cervix is thought to retain some "memory" so that it dilates more quickly. Also, as mentioned above, often you are already dilated before labour begins so that you are starting off ahead of the game. Many women will remember how to push effectively, and so are more efficient at pushing the baby out. In fact, for first babies the second stage lasts about an hour, while for subsequent babies, it may only take about 20 minutes.

While for most women having their second child labour and delivery are shorter, this is not true for everyone. Sometimes if the baby is larger, or the head is positioned in a way that makes delivery more difficult, the labour will be longer or may even require a caesarean section. It is important to be prepared.

Coping with the pain of labour

There is no doubt that for most women, labour is accompanied by a significant amount of pain. While childbirth classes can be very helpful for teaching techniques to lessen the pain, many women prefer to receive a form of pain relief at some point during labour. The two options for pain relief are either analgesic medications, which dampen or reduce the pain, or regional anaesthetics, such as an epidural. An epidural is a type of regional anaesthesia in which drugs are injected into the space around the membranes that cover the lower part of the spinal cord, relieving pain below the level of the injection. This provides an excellent form a pain relief in labour and many women today opt for an epidural for optimal pain relief.

For your first pregnancy, you may have wanted to experience as "natural" a delivery as possible, perhaps even without any pain medication or anaesthesia. We have had many patients who tell us, after receiving an epidural, "Why did I wait so long? What was I thinking?" If your first birth left you feeling that labour was more painful and difficult than you would care to experience again, choosing either pain medications or regional anaesthesia may be a good option for you the second time around.

The good news is that it really does not prolong active labour, although it may make the second stage take a little longer. If, however, you laboured the first time without any pain medication or anaesthesia and felt that it was the right choice for you, you may choose to do the same this time around. Or, if you had pain medications, you may now feel you want to deliver more naturally since pain medications do have their drawbacks. An epidural requires continuous fetal heart monitoring and a drip to supply fluids and some women having one suffer from backache or find it hard to adopt a comfortable position. Pethidine can make you feel sick and forgetful.

Repeat episiotomy

A minor surgical procedure, an episiotomy is an incision made along the perineum (region between the vagina and rectum) to enlarge the vaginal opening just prior to the birth of the baby. There are two types: a median incision extends along the midline towards the rectum and a mediolateral incision veers off towards one side. Interestingly the use of episiotomy varies significantly between countries, being about 14% in the UK, 25% in the US, 1% in Sweden and 80% in Argentina.

There are some benefits to having an episiotomy rather than risking a tear: it may enable a faster delivery of the baby in the case of a worrisome fetal heart rate tracing and it is easier to repair than a tear and heals more quickly. It is controversial whether it decreases the incidence of more severe lacerations.

Some potential negatives to episiotomy include increased postpartum pain, greater blood loss and a possible increased risk of a laceration in a subsequent pregnancy. These days, most midwives do not routinely perform an episiotomy, but make the decision at the actual time of delivery.

If you had an episiotomy the first time, it does not necessarily mean that you will have an episiotomy again. In fact, because the vaginal tissues tend to be more stretched, episiotomy is less likely to be performed. If you were able to avoid an episiotomy the first time, you will be likely to avoid it again (unless some unforeseen complication arises, like a drop in the rate of the fetal heart beat, difficulty delivering your baby's shoulder, etc.).

EPISIOTOMY CUTS

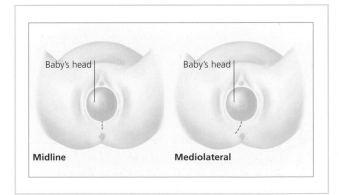

Baby's head

Baby's head

Midline

Mediolateral

Vaginal birth after a caesarean (VBAC)

Trends in performing a repeat caesarean section or allowing a woman a trial of labour after a prior caesarean section keep on changing. Many years ago, the prevailing thought was "Once a caesarean, always a caesarean". In the 1990s things changed and a trial of VBAC became more common. In the early 2000's, as new data emerged about the risks of uterine rupture after caesarean section, particularly for those women undergoing induction of labour with certain types of medications, the emphasis changed again. Repeat caesarean sections became more frequent while VBACs began to decline. Today, doctors and women are again beginning to focus on VBAC as a good alternative to elective repeat caesarean sections.

Benefits and risks

There are a number of each. The medical benefits of a VBAC may include a shorter length of hospital stay, an easier recovery, a lower chance of developing a blood clot in the leg or lung, a reduced risk of needing a blood transfusion and lower rates of fever, wound infection or infection within the uterus post-delivery. Also, for those women who are planning a large family, having a successful VBAC will mean that they would, most likely, be able to have vaginal deliveries in the future, which would reduce the chance of scar tissue forming after each caesarean delivery.

In addition to the medical benefits, there may be psychological or emotional benefits as well. If a woman wanted to experience a vaginal delivery the first time around and did not, a VBAC can give her the emotional fulfillment and the joy of a new experience.

While there certainly are clear medical benefits to VBAC, there are also risks that you need to take into account if you are considering a trial of labour.

The most worrisome and important risk is that of uterine rupture, where the scar on your uterus opens up and causes problems for either you or your baby. A less serious condition, uterine dehiscence, may prevent you having a vaginal birth now or in the future (see box).

You may want to consider having a trial of labour if you have had only one prior caesarean section with a low transverse incision, have no other uterine

UTERINE CAESAREAN INCISIONS

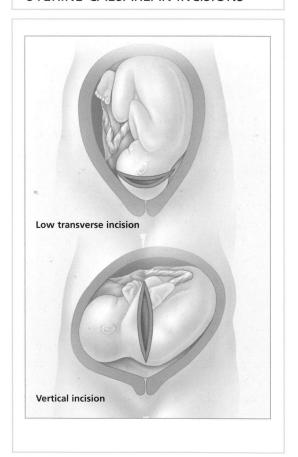

Low transverse incision

Vertical incision

scars from prior surgeries, do not have any other obstetric indications for a caesarean section (placenta praevia or a fetus that is not head down, for example), are in a hospital setting where there are anaesthetists and an operating room immediately available in case of emergencies, and you completely understand all of the risks mentioned above.

Bear in mind that the type of scar on your abdomen does not necessarily reflect the type of scar on your uterus. Your caregiver should have a copy of your notes from your first caesarean section and so will be able to counsel you about the risks.

Keep in mind that while VBAC for most women is very safe, there are some rare risks. While fetal death occurs more often with VBAC than with repeat caesarean delivery, it is still extremely rare. Maternal mortality is extremely rare with either type of delivery.

What are the chances that if you attempt a VBAC you will be successful? Well, you will be happy to know that the odds are in your favour. In general, the success rates of VBAC are about 60–80 per cent if certain factors are taken into consideration (see box, page 92).

How your labour is managed may differ slightly from that of women who have not had a prior caesarean section. Delivery should take place in a hospital rather than at home so there is immediate access to an operating room and anaesthesia. Your baby's heart rate and your uterine contractions will probably be continuously monitored. If oxytocin is necessary it will be used cautiously, and certain mediations used to induce the labour, such as prostaglandin E1, will not be used as this is associated with uterine hyperstimulation, which increases the risk of uterine rupture. There is a safer alternative, prostaglandin E2, also known as Prostin, dinoprostone, or Prepidil.

Arranging to have a VBAC

Because it is a contentious situation, not every consultant or hospital is in favour. It is therefore

---

MORE**ABOUT**   uterine rupture and dehiscence

If you have a VBAC and successfully deliver vaginally, your doctor will check the wall of the uterus after delivery to see if the uterine scar from the prior caesarean section is intact. If it is found to be open, it is called a dehiscence. This may also occur if you try a VBAC and end up needing a caesarean section. If at the time of the repeat caesarean your doctor notices that the scar has separated, again it is called a dehiscence, and you will be cautioned that you should not attempt a VBAC in the future.

If you have what is called a uterine rupture, the opening of the scar will have resulted in complications, most commonly a drop in the fetal heart rate during attempted labour. In addition, uterine rupture can cause you to bleed excessively, although this is quite a rare complication. The

chances of uterine rupture depend partly on the type of initial incision made during the first caesarean section. Most commonly a transverse (horizontal) incision is made in the lower portion of the uterus, and this has the lowest risk of rupture (0.2-1.5 per cent). The risk of rupture is higher with a "classical", or vertical (up-and-down) incision or a T-shaped incision on the uterus, with rupture rates of about 4-9 per cent. This type of incision is more likely (but not necessarily) to have been made if you delivered prematurely, had a placenta praevia or the baby was lying across your uterus (transverse lie).

advisable to do some research ahead of time and to know up front what you're dealing with than to arrive for your birth and be disappointed.

Check with the providers in your area to be sure that a VBAC is permitted. Some hospitals still refuse to allow this process. Call your local hospital and ask for its policies regarding VBACs, as well as its current caesarean rate. Talk to other pregnant women you know that have had VBACs and ask if they know of doctors who support the process. Read a variety of books about VBAC, and arm yourself with current statistics regarding both VBAC and caesarean sections.

Discuss your preference for a VBAC with your midwife, doctor and hospital. One or the other may try to discourage you, or they simply may make you aware of the statistics regarding VBACs and allow you to make your own choice. Either way, try to keep in mind that this is your birth, not theirs. Do the best you can to ensure that you get to make the decision, while taking into account their expert advice.

When making the decision with your caregiver whether or not to undergo a VBAC, it is also important to consider how many children you desire. If you are planning a large family, you may be more inclined to try a VBAC, so that you are not committed to multiple caesarean sections and their risks (see page 93). On the other hand, if you only plan on having two children, you might want to have a scheduled repeat caesarean and avoid any possible risks of rupture.

7 situations that are more likely to result in a successful VBAC

1 You have had a vaginal delivery or a successful VBAC in the past.

2 Your prior caesarean section was performed for a non-recurring cause, like a breech presentation or placenta praevia.

3 Your prior caesarean section was performed either prior to or early in labour (not after full dilatation).

4 Your current labour occurs spontaneously (it is not induced) and your waters break on their own.

5 You are not put on a drip to speed the labour up.

6 The baby's heartbeat is monitored regularly with a pinard (midwife's stethoscope) or a Doppler (sonicaid).

7 You keep moving around and try to stay upright.

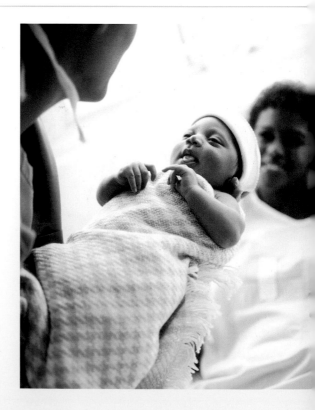

Caesarean section

Circumstances can arise, which necessitate a caesarean delivery the second time around. If you were trying for a vaginal delivery again but require a caesarean, you may find that you feel frustrated, disappointed or a failure in some way. While this is understandable, remember that the ultimate goal is the safe delivery of your child and your own health and safety. Caesarean sections are either performed electively (planned ahead of time), are unplanned in labour or are emergencies (see box).

Repeat cesarean section

If you have made the decision to have a planned repeat caesarean section, the next thing you should think about is picking a delivery date. For the most part, the decision should be based on gestational age. It appears that the best outcome for babies follows a planned repeat caesarean at around 39 to 40 weeks. Delivery at this gestational age is associated with the lowest risk of newborn complications (respiratory problems, admissions to the neonatal intensive care unit and stillbirth) and the less chance of you going into labour. If you have the kind of scar on your uterus that is associated with a greater risk of uterine rupture (see page 91), it might be advisable to be delivered earlier.

Risks of more than two

If you are having your third caesarean section, you are facing issues that require some thought and planning by your doctors. Multiple caesarean sections increase the risk for placenta accreta (the placenta being abnormally implanted into the uterus) as well as risks of more scar tissue, greater chances of bleeding that require a hysterectomy, or having an injury to the bladder or bowel during the surgery. Your doctors may take extra precautions, like having extra blood ready for transfusions.

TYPE OF CAESAREAN DELIVERY

A planned caesarean will be done if:
- The baby is very large (estimated fetal weight greater than 4500 grams in a woman who has diabetes and greater than 5000 grams in a womean without diabetes)
- Placenta or vasa praevia (the placenta or umbilical cord lie over the cervix) is present
- Fetal presentation is transverse lie or breech
- Previous uterine surgery (removal of fibroids, caesarean section, etc.) was done
- Twins, triplets or more babies are expected
- Certain maternal medical conditions – heart and inflammatory bowel disease – are present
- The woman wishes

An unplanned but non-emergency caesarean will be done if:
- Labour stops progressing or progresses slowly because either the baby is thought to be too big to fit through the birth canal or the position of the baby's head makes vaginal delivery unlikely
- Fetal monitoring suggests that the baby is not tolerating labour
- Maternal medical conditions – pre-eclampsia, maternal heart disease, etc. – worsen

An emergency caesarean will be carried out if:
- There is a prolonged drop in the baby's heart rate
- Excessive bleeding occurs
- The baby's umbilical cord or a fetal part prolapses or protrudes through the cervix

Involving your child and partner

Many women who chose to have their babies at home do so because they feel they will be happier, have more support and be better able to cope with their families around them.

Children in at the delivery

As well as at home, it also may be possible to have your child with you if you deliver in hospital or in a midwife unit. But as well as ascertaining whether the hospital or unit will allow your child to be present, and even if you plan to have your birth at home, it's also important to consider some other factors when deciding whether your child should see the birth. Things to consider are:

• The age of your child;
• The maturity of your child;
• The interest your child has in seeing the birth.

If your child is less than four years old, he may be too young to appreciate the experience, but more importantly, he may be scared by what is happening. If you are in pain, bleeding or have a drip attached to your arm, it may frighten your child rather than making him feel a part of the process in a positive way. If your child is older, it is reasonable to ask him if he wants to be in the room.

If your child expresses real interest and enthusiasm in being present, then you can sit down and explain to him exactly what he should expect. It is a good idea if you are delivering in hospital, to give him a picture of what the room looks like and where you will be. You will also want to explain how you will be examined and how the baby will actually be born. Make sure you let him know that sometimes unexpected things can happen, and that it is possible you could be taken to the hospital from home, or if already in hospital, be wheeled to a different room to have the baby by caesarean section.

Your child may benefit from seeing pictures in books or watching an educational movie about the whole birth process. Also, when the big event happens, remember that labour can take a long time, so be prepared by making sure he has plenty of activities to keep him busy.

Keep in mind that no matter how mature or excited your child seems, he may not ultimately react the way you anticipate. Sometimes the delivery room is too intense and scary even for a very mature child. You should have an additional adult available to take him out of the room if he feels uncomfortable, and also reassure him that you will not be disappointed if this happens.

Second-time birth partner

From the beginning, it will not be surprising if your partner seems a little more casual and laid-back about the pregnancy. He may not "ooh" and "aah" each time you feel fetal movement, and be less interested in reading pregnancy books the second time around! You may notice he doesn't make every antenatal appointment, or attend every antenatal class. This is not unusual, and you yourself may be less preoccupied with pregnancy this time around. You may miss an occasional antenatal visit, or be a little less vigilant about what you are eating or how you are preparing for the new baby. This is all normal, and in fact, often continues after the baby is born. The good part about this is that there is oftenmore of a feeling of relaxation, and less anxiety. This may also continue into the delivery room.

If your partner seems less attentive, and more calm, it doesn't mean that he is less interested, or is not as excited about having the baby as the first time, but just that he has been through it before and is more relaxed.

Baby blues and depression

Pregnant women and their families and friends assume that the postpartum period is a time filled with utter joy, elation and happiness. Unfortunately the reality is that up to 20 to 80 per cent of women experience either some degree of baby blues or depression, and half of these are women having their second or third child.

Baby blues are usually short-lived, and associated with mood swings, anxiety, difficulty sleeping, and crying spells. About 40 to 80 per cent of women develop these mood changes, usually about two to three days after delivery, and they usually resolve within two weeks.

Postnatal depression, on the other hand, occurs in about 10 per cent of mothers, with a lifetime risk up to 25 per cent. This means that if you did not have it the first time, you may still be at risk for having it in a second pregnancy. Some symptoms to look out for are inability to sleep (even when your baby is asleep), poor appetite, rapid weight loss, profound lack of energy, anxiety, feeling overwhelmed and unable to care for the baby, feeling inadequate as a mother, not bonding to the baby and not feeling any sense of pleasure or joy when being with your baby. Some women experience thoughts about harming themselves or their babies, but rarely disclose these thoughts.

Seeking help

If you feel any of the symptoms described above, it is important to speak to your healthcare provider. If you are suffering from depression, there are several approaches to improving the situation, including medications, getting adequate sleep, psychotherapy or marital therapy if that is where the problem lies. Most important, is to remember not to feel guilty about this. Having postnatal depression or the blues does not mean that you love your child any less. In fact, by seeking help, you are doing your best to not only take care of yourself but your family as well.

Postnatal depression risks

Women at higher risk for depression include those:

- With a stressful life in the last year;
- Experiencing marital conflict;
- Living without a partner;
- Whose pregnancies are unplanned;
- Who have a history of depression (either when non-pregnant or with the last pregnancy)
- Who have stress issues related to child care;
- With a perceived lack of support from family and friends;
- Having a family psychiatric history.

A thought for your partner

Postnatal depression has long been thought of as a condition that only affects mums but researchers are now starting to take it seriously as an issue for dads. A recent study of more than 8,000 fathers in the UK found that eight weeks after the birth, one in 25 was suffering postnatal depression, compared to one in 10 mothers. Of course, just about everyone will experience a few rough weeks, but if the feelings continue, a depressed father can be a devastating blow for the family, to the point where he leaves the home or becomes suicidal. It's also been suggested that a depressed father has a particularly bad effect on the development of his sons, as boys appear to be influenced from a very early age by paternal behaviour.

The big problem for men is that they are much less likely than women to ask for help. So, if you suspect your partner may be suffering, have a word with him and, if necessary, your doctor.

Getting back in shape

How fast you start to regain your pre-pregnancy figure will depend on a number of factors including the type of birth you had and whether you breastfeed your baby.

If you had an uncomplicated vaginal birth, you can be back home within 24 hours. The community midwife will visit you at home and help you to care for yourself and your baby. After the first few weeks, a health visitor – a trained nurse and midwife whose specialty is infants and young children up to school entry – will help with care.

If you had a caesarean delivery, you will be in hospital longer – about five to seven days. Although the staff will help you become mobile as quickly as possible, you will need to take things very easy the first few weeks.

Caring for your scar

By the time you leave hospital, your abdomen should be feeling less tender. If you are still in pain, keep taking pain relief to keep it under control and allow you to keep moving. Your sutures or stitches will be removed, leaving you with a scar. This may consist of a hard ridge along the incision, but it will gradually soften as it heals. The area may feel quite numb, which is natural, but the numbness will reduce as healing continues. You may, however, be left with some numbness directly around the scar for a long time. Some women never get all the feeling back in the area around their scars.

You will be advised on how to clean the area and to check for redness or swelling. It's important to familiarise yourself with your scar so that you will recognise if it starts looking abnormal. If you feel discomfort, try placing a heated pad or a warm, moist towel against the area.

Afterpains

Contractions post birth enable your uterus to return to its pre-pregnant size and location. You probably didn't notice these cramps much after your first delivery, but they can be quite painful after a second delivery – some women require medication – and usually get worse with each successive pregnancy. This is mainly due to poorer muscle tone as a result of another pregnancy and delivery. The cramping will be at its most intense one or two days after giving birth and it can take up to six weeks or longer for your uterus to return to its normal size. Breastfeeding can bring on these cramps or make them more intense because your baby's sucking triggers the release of the hormone oxytocin, which in turn causes contractions. This is why breastfeeding is advised to help your uterus return to its pre-pregnant condition.

There are some things you can do to try to help you cope with the pains but if the cramping doesn't ease up after a few days or the pain becomes unbearable, call your caregiver. It could be a sign of infection or another problem that requires medical attention.

HEALTH FIRST	caesarean incision

If the scar becomes painful, red or swollen, or there is an unusual discharge, seek medical attention. If the bleeding from the incision stops and then starts again, or if it soaks more than one dressing every hour, or turns bright red, discuss with your doctor or midwife urgently.

- Urinate often, even if you don't feel the urge to go, because a full bladder displaces the uterus so it can't contract as well as it should;
- Spend some time lying face down with a pillow under your lower belly;
- Gentlly massage your lower belly;
- Take some ibuprofen.

Fitness routine

If you delivered by caesarean section rather than delivering vaginally, your doctors may advise you to wait for six weeks before resuming exercise. Also, if you didn't exercise regularly before, you will probably be slower to start a regime now. But bear in mind, it's never too late; the sooner you get yourself into shape, the better you will feel.

Because many of the physical changes of pregnancy persist up to 6-12 weeks after the delivery, your post-pregnancy exercise routines should be started gradually. Keep in mind, of course, the shape you were in during your pregnancy. If you continued to run five miles a day during the pregnancy, you can probably resume that pretty quickly after delivery.

Women having their second child often find that it takes a little longer to get back into their jeans this time around. The abdominal wall has been stretched again, and it may be harder to tighten up the abdominal muscles this time. Also, if not all the baby weight gained for a first child was lost, there will be even more to lose this time.

Your pelvic floor muscles may also need toning as shown by your finding it difficult to control your bladder if you laugh or move suddenly.

Try to find the time to get into an exercise routine. Even taking your baby for long walks in nice weather is helpful.

Postnatal perineal exercise

As important as it is to keep your pelvic muscles in shape while you are pregnant, it's even more important once you've given birth. When you've mastered the exercise on page 56, and as you gain greater control over your pelvic muscles, you can try this additional exercise.

There are individual bands of muscle which surround each of the three openings – anus, vagina and bladder – and each band of muscle is capable of being contracted in isolation. Try to squeeze the muscles around the back passage (anus) then release. Now try and squeeze the muscles around the vagina (the muscles you use during sex) and release. Finally, squeeze the muscles you use when you go to the

Sometimes its easier to locate with your perineal muscles when you adopt an all-fours position.

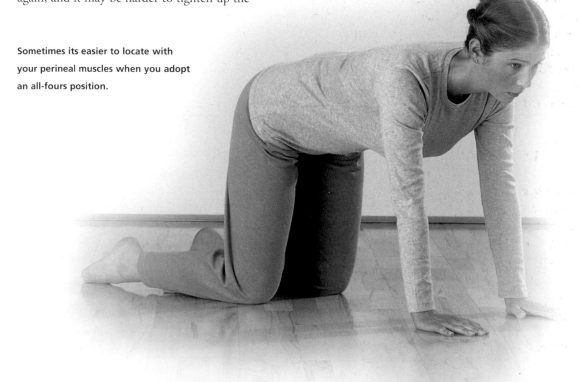

toilet to pass urine and release. Practice "back, middle, front" until you have gained full control over each individual ring of muscle. Now try and hold each band of muscle for one minute before releasing and moving on to the next. Do several sets of this exercise at least three times a day.

Sensible eating

If you are breastfeeding, you will require extra calories and liquids (see page 49). While breastfeeding can help your tummy return to its pre-pregnant shape, because it makes the uterus contract and uses up more calories, your breasts will remain quite large and you may not regain your pre-pregnancy weight until you stop breastfeeding. Although some women do it sooner, many women take 10 to 14 months to get back to their pre-pregnancy body weight, stamina and strength.

If you are bottle feeding, you don't need any extra calories but you need to eat a varied diet to ensure you get the nutrients you need to recover from the birth and cope with broken nights. Lots of fruit, vegetables, lean meat, poultry, fish and beans as well as carbohydrates such as bread and pasta will help you get back in shape.

Don't be tempted to go on a crash diet or take slimming pills. They can make it more difficult for you to lose weight in the long term and may make you feel very tired.

Your postnatal check

About six weeks after the birth, you will be seen either in hospital or by your GP to ensure that you are recovering as expected. If you have had a caesarean, you may have an additional check at 12 weeks after the birth.

Among the checks carried out:
- you may be weighed;
- your blood pressure tested;
- your urine tested.

You may be offered an examination to see whether your stitches or incision scar have healed, your uterus is back to its normal size, and all the muscles used during labour and delivery are returning to their normal condition.

If you haven't had a cervical smear test in the past three years, you may be advised to have one about three months post delivery. Similarly, if you are not immune to German measles (rubella) and have not received an immunisation prior to leaving hospital, you will be offered one now.

Contraception will be discussed again (as it should have been when you left hospital), and you may now be able to be fitted with a cap or diaphragm or IUD (intrauterine device). If you've completed your family, you might want to discuss tubal ligation or vasectomy with your doctor.

Your doctor will want to know whether you still have any vaginal discharge, whether your periods have resumed and if you're feeling very tired, low or depressed (see page 95).

Make sure you tell your doctor if you are having trouble holding your urine, are experiencing a lot of wind or are soiling yourself.

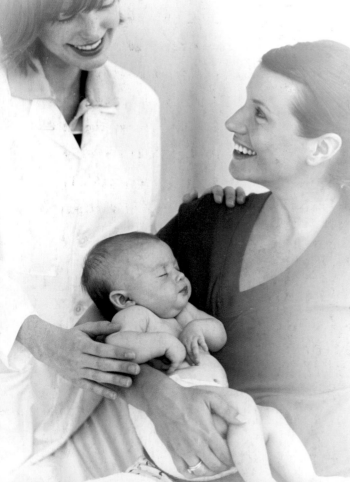

SECOND TIME PARENT

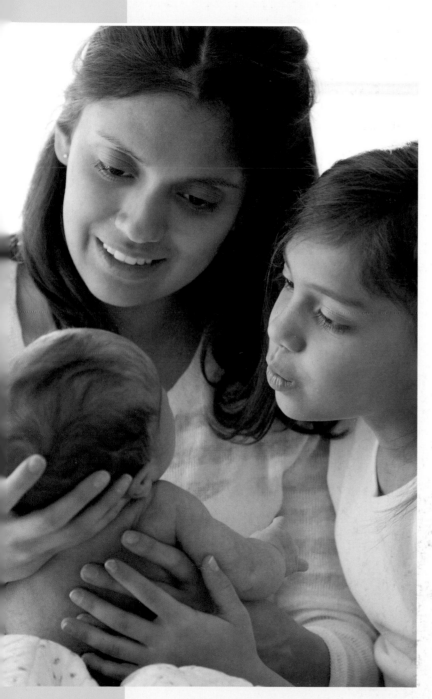

At last your baby has arrived and with him or her a change in family dynamics. You'll probably be amazed at how quickly your love expands to embrace this new family member and how this gives you some of the strength you need to cope with your added responsibilities. Although it won't all be plain sailing in future, particularly if your existing child isn't as thrilled as you with having a new brother or sister, you'll soon find that a two or even three-child family is defined by the old adage – "the more the merrier"!

Immediate concerns

Whatever else you are worried about, it shouldn't be whether you can manage the day-to-day routines. There's nothing like first-hand experience of caring for a baby to build up childcare skills and you probably cannot believe how much you learned with your first born. You established procedures and routines for many of the daily tasks that initially baffled you, you kept your baby comforted, amused and stimulated, and you probably even managed occasional free time to put your feet up and relax. Although life as a parent of one child is hectic and challenging – and won't get easier, only different, as she grows older – your confidence has risen and, with a bit of luck, you feel ready and able to cope with your second. And you are. But don't be surprised if things don't go as smoothly as you might expect.

The psychological and physical needs of your second baby are essentially the same as those of your first; for example, she will need to be loved, cared for, stimulated and to feel secure, etc. – these are universal needs of every child. But each baby is a unique individual with her own characteristics, personality and way of interacting with the world around her, so, in order to best meet these universal needs, your response may have to vary. For instance, your first born might have been easily soothed simply by being held in your arms; the basic act of bringing her close to you could have been enough to stop her tears. In contrast, your second baby might take much longer to calm down; perhaps she will need you to talk to her, rock her and give her another feed before she will be able to settle and relax. Or maybe she won't be so easily amused as

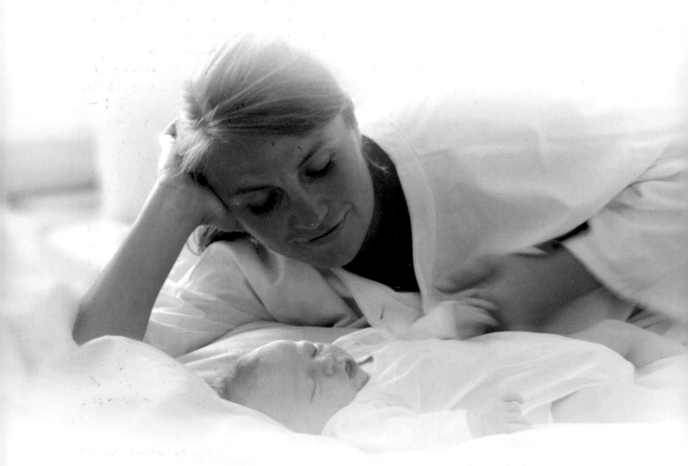

Bonding is vital to future success

A child who fails to form an emotional attachment with at least one adult by the time she has reached the age of three or four is likely to have difficulty forming relationships with others throughout her life. She may suffer from low self-esteem and have lower educational achievements at every stage of school.

your eldest, requiring more input from you before she starts showing interest in toys. You should resist the temptation to assume that "one size fits all" when it comes to parenting; you may be very surprised to discover how very different your second experience of parenting is from your first.

Your immediate concerns second time around will be establishing a strong emotional bond with your baby, finding out how to best meet her feeding and sleeping needs and ensuring you get enough rest for yourself. These will remain top priorities but as you'll soon have two children trying to grab your attention at the same time – with each one convinced that she is more important than her sibling – you will have to learn how to balance their competing psychological needs. So, you've still got lots to do, despite all the parenting experiences you have had up to now.

Bonding with your second baby

You probably have formed a close, emotional attachment with your first baby and this provides her with a sense of love, comfort and security. It's also important for her future, as the quality of this lasting attachment will have the greatest effect on her subsequent psychological development. With your second baby, bonding is just as important; she also needs that warm loving relationship with you and you need it as well in order to feel positive

about yourself. There is something wonderful about knowing that your baby loves you, feels safe with you and is secure when you hold her.

The chances are that you'll bond as easily with baby number two as you did with baby number one, yet some factors present in your life now could influence the relationship with your second child. One is that you already have a baby you love and you will instinctively compare the next one to her; the results of that comparison can affect your feelings towards your second born. Then there's the time element. With your first baby, you were able to devote most of your waking hours towards her without any pressure to divert your attention elsewhere. That undoubtedly helped facilitate the bonding process. Now you have to care for two, which means splitting your time in ways that you didn't have to previously. In addition, raising two young children at the same time saps both physical and psychological energy and can make you very tired. The net result is that some parents have to work harder at building an emotional attachment with their second baby than they did with their first.

Bear in mind that bonding is rarely instantaneous. It is not a magical all-or-nothing process that must occur in an instant or not at all. Even if you didn't immediately fall in love with your first baby and may be guilt-ridden about it and possibly afraid it will take even longer with your second baby, you are worrying unnecessarily. Psychological investigations have revealed that at least 40 per cent of perfectly normal mothers take a minimum of a week – and often months – to feel that their babies are really theirs.

The truth is that instant bonding is far from the minds of many parents just after the births of their second children. On seeing their baby right after the delivery, they may have thoughts such as "Gosh, my first baby didn't look so bruised and ugly", "I hope I can manage with two because I find managing one hard enough", or "Will I be a good parent to him because I've heard that boys are so much more difficult than girls". Doubts and anxieties such as these are perfectly normal with a second baby, and are nothing to feel guilty about. They will soon pass

6 ways to get closer

1 **Talk to your baby as often as you can** Even though your baby doesn't understand the words you say, she loves to hear the familiar tone of your voice and quickly learns to associate it with comfort, safety, security and love. You can speak to her, for example, while changing her or feeding her or while taking her out in her buggy during the day. Through interacting together in this way, you and your second baby will gradually get to know each other. Your comfort and ease in each other's company will steadily increase with each passing day and this will enhance your emotional connection.

2 **Use feeding times to establish eye contact** Whether you bottle-feed or breastfeed your baby, look lovingly into your baby's eyes while you hold her during a feed. Research has shown that when a baby is born her eyes focus at a distance approximately seven to nine inches (18–23 cm) away from her nose – this is almost exactly the distance between your face and hers when holding her as she takes her feed. In other words, she is pre-programmed to see your face. Smile at her lovingly and look deep into her eyes. The bond between you will become stronger.

3 **Soothe your baby when she is upset** It's never easy calming a crying baby, and particularly so if your older child was a more settled baby. You may feel frustrated by this baby's screams and tears and unsure why, in contrast to your first born, she seems to cry all the time. Try different soothing techniques; as with your first, you'll gradually get to know what this baby's cries mean, and the best way to ease her distress. Don't give up just because it's different this time round. Keep trying different approaches until one works.

4 **Try and reflect her emotions** Bonding requires you to become attuned to your baby's feelings, to understand what she's thinking at the time, and to show her that you have achieved this level of insight. So when she smiles at you, smile back twice as broadly. When she is upset, tell her that you can see she is upset and try to comfort her. When she is interested in something (perhaps a toy or household object), help her play with it. The more you accurately reflect her feelings, the more connected she will feel with you.

5 **Take pride in her achievements** What is so wonderful about the first years of life is that your baby makes terrific progress. There are so many changes in terms of physical prowess, vocalisations and emotional and social skills. Some parents find that they are not so excited with all these developmental steps when it comes to a second baby – almost as if the novelty has worn off to some extent. Yet the formation of emotional bonds is enhanced when you take delight in your baby's achievements, both large and small. Your praise and pleasure at, for example, her ability to sit up on her own without support, lets her know that you love and value her.

6 **Keep a baby record** As well as demonstrating this through your words and caring gestures, you can take practical actions. For instance, you can record each special event, each progression in development in a baby record book. That's also a good place to attach mementos such as a lock of her hair. Another way is to simply keep a photograph book, which documents her week by week, or month by month, changes. These methods help focus your attention on her progress and achievement, and, in a couple of years, she'll take great delight in pouring over them with you.

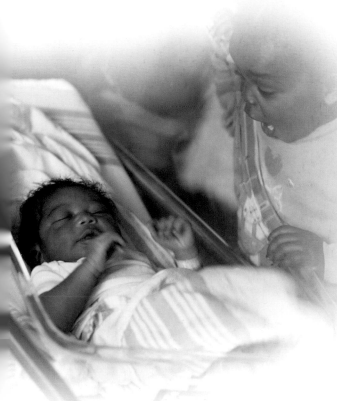

Nor should you worry if you aren't able to hold your second baby the moment she is born (for instance, because she is delivered by an emergency caesarean section while you were under a general anaesthetic) whereas your firstborn was in your arms within seconds of the birth. After all, it's only in the past 30 years or so that mothers who give birth in hospital have been allowed physical contact with their new babies; prior to that, a baby was kept in a nursery and contact was only allowed at feeding time, and yet nearly all of them bonded with their mothers.

Helping the bonding process

It is perfectly normal for a mother of a second baby to have some self-doubts about how much she will love her second baby and about how good a parent she will be to this one, even though she has a proven track record with her first baby. The awesome responsibility of raising two, instead of just one, can unsteady the most self-assured parent. So get involved straight away. The best technique for strengthening your bond with your second baby is by tackling the basic challenges of babycare – feeding, cleaning, changing and comforting. These activities can seem mundane yet they bring you and your baby in frequent, close physical and emotional contact. (See also box.)

After returning to work

As the months pass, you might decide it's time to get back to work, to pick up your career again where you left off after this temporary break to have your second baby. Almost certainly, though, you will have mixed feelings about this.

On the one hand, the thought of being back at work, mixing with colleagues once again and having professional challenges (and perhaps of escaping from the routine of babycare) may make you excited. On the other hand, the prospect of spending each day away from both your delightful young children might fill you with despair as will worry about keeping the bond with your children strong. And if you are returning to work solely for financial reasons and would much rather continue in

as your confidence as a mother of two grows with experience. Bonding is usually a gradual process.

And then there are all your pre-birth expectations to deal with. Some mums tacitly assume that their second will look like their first, have the same nature and be as talented – in other words, they are not expecting any significant differences between their two children.

There is also the baby's gender to consider. Everyone has his or her own (often unspoken) preferences to have a second baby of a specific gender (either to match the one they have, so that, say, each has a brother, or to complement the child they have, so that there is a boy and a girl in the family).

Therefore, if your prenatal hopes and expectations about similarities and differences between your first born and second born are not met, you may feel emotionally confused, perhaps even disappointed, when your second baby arrives. The chances are, however, that you'll very quickly start to relate to her because of her unique qualities, and you'll form an attachment as easily with her as you did with your first baby.

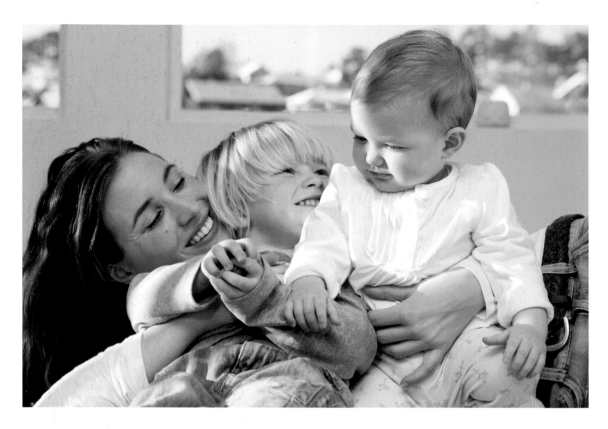

your role as principal carer for your children, each day getting to know them better and strengthening the emotional connection between you, then you may worry that the warm relationship you have with them will suffer.

With a little effort and planning, however, there is no reason why you can't keep a healthy psychological connection between you and both your children even though you have returned to the workforce. What matters isn't the amount of time you spend with your children but the quality of the time you spend with them. Babies who spend all day with grumpy, hostile, unloving mothers are less likely to bond than those who only a spend time at the start and the end of each day with loving, attentive, caring mothers. If you have a positive approach, valuing those precious moments together, then that adds to the bonding process.

You will need to manage your time more effectively, so that you spend as much time with your children as possible. Do what you can to match your free time in the morning and evenings with your babies' individual eating and sleeping routines. If, for instance, your second baby is usually asleep when you arrive home but normally wakes up an hour later, use that first hour for playing with your elder child. And if she is awake before you leave in the morning, then try to plan to have that time with her.

Instead of worrying about how lonely your children are with you back at work, enjoy the times that you do have with them. Talk to them, play with them, cuddle them, sing to them, wash them, change them – in fact, do whatever you like as long as you are relaxed and happy in their company. These shared, loving moments keeps the bonding process alive and well. Try to relax, and do what you can to ignore distractions such as ringing doorbells and telephones when you are with your children. Ring-fence these periods and have fun, without feeling guilty.

There is no reason to assume that your second baby will lose out psychologically by your return to work when she is still young or that her attachment to you will suffer, even if you didn't return to work after your first birth. There is ample research evidence that confirms babies in this situation thrive normally – assuming there is good quality childcare while mum is out during the day and that mother and baby have a high quality relationship when they are together.

One of the disappointments that many mothers experience when they return to work soon after their second baby arrives is that they miss out on some of those enjoyable moments spent with their baby, like the time he gave his first smile or first grabbed for the toy in front of him. Not being there for those precious events, those endless "firsts" that make caring for a baby so enjoyable, can create pangs of jealousy, longing and guilt. But it needn't be like that if you return to work and leave your baby with someone else during the day. Just make a point of spending a few minutes with your carer at the end of each working day to discuss all the happenings of the day. That way you'll be able to keep up with your baby's progress even though you don't actually experience each new progression personally.

You may have the opportunity to consider the possibility of returning to work while your partner becomes the main carer – more and more dads are either taking advantage of paternity leave soon after their babies are born, or are giving up work altogether as their partners earn as much (if not more) than them.

If your partner is a willing participant in such an arrangement, that may suit everyone. You'll be able to pick up your career where you left off, knowing that your second baby is in the care of her competent, loving father rather than in the hands of a paid child-minder. Of course, both you and your partner have to be in full agreement about this or resentment and confusion could develop in your relationship. Of course, whichever way you organise your working lives after the arrival of your second baby, it will be more successful and satisfactory if you and your partner have discussed it fully with each other and are in agreement.

In the end, it all comes down to balancing need against choice. If you feel that you have to go back to work because of economic and financial constraints, but you would actually prefer to raise your baby yourself at home, there is a risk of resentment and bitterness at having to take on a role you'd rather not.

Perhaps, though, the situation will not be as cut and dried as it initially appears. For instance, you could decide to forego the additional income from full-time work and instead settle for a part-time income. Or you and your partner could decide to accept the financial strain of one of you staying at home to raise your second baby without using a carer. Think all the different options through very carefully before deciding on a course of action.

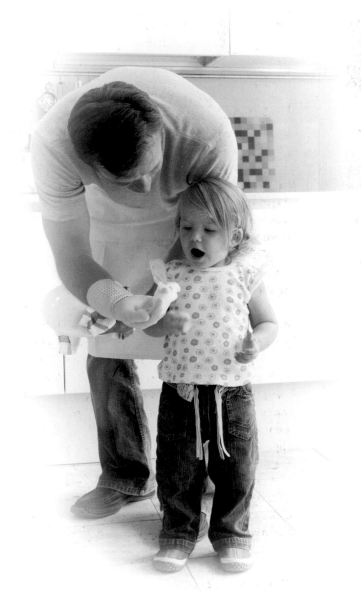

Getting through the early days

Managing two children, one of whom is a young baby, requires planning and prioritisation – you'll find that time and energy are in short supply, and that you simply can't run your life the way you did before your second baby arrived. Caring for two is more demanding than caring for one, even though you are more experienced this time round.

Your priorities

There are two essential interrelated priorities for you personally at this stage. The first priority is to ensure you get ample rest – looking after two young children is physically and emotionally demanding. Of course, you'll never have as much sleep as you'd like, but that doesn't mean you have to walk around in an exhausted stupor, lurching from one feed to another, one changing and bathing routine to

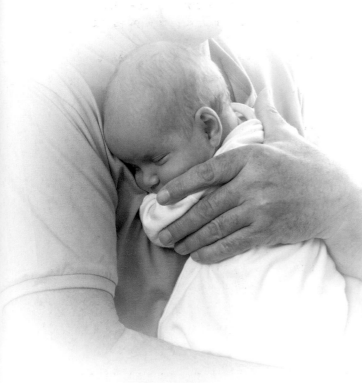

another, or from one tidying up to another. Take naps whenever you can. Encourage your first-born and your second baby to have a midday sleep at the same time – you never know, it might actually work out that way. And if they do nod off at the same time, have a rest yourself, even if you don't manage to actually fall asleep. Plan your social life sensibly. You have nothing to prove. Go out with your partner and friends when you feel like it and when you have someone to look after your kids. But there may be times when you might just prefer to crawl into bed and leave the socialising to someone else.

The second priority is to ensure that you get help from others, where possible. Your partner, best friend, extended family or neighbours are all potential sources of support. Don't try to convince yourself that you should cope with everything on your own – even if you can, you'll still benefit from help. Whether it's a case of your friend minding both children for half an hour, your partner taking his turn to give a night feed to your second baby, or grandma taking your youngest out to the park for an hour when your older child is at preschool, every little bit helps. It might not occur to others that you would want that sort of support, so be prepared to ask. You may be pleasantly surprised by the positive responses you receive.

Try to have a structure to your day, especially during the first year of your second baby's life. Plan out a rough schedule of activities, including meals, bathing, play, daytime naps and bedtime. Think about your children's natural physical cycles in terms of eating, sleeping, concentration and wakefulness, and arrange activities to take this into account. For example, if you know your second baby is very unsettled after lunch, that's clearly not the time to go to your local shopping centre with her. The chances are you won't be able to stick to everything on your list, but it will provide some structure to your day. You'll feel more in control, less stressed and less tired.

Strategies and schedules

The biggest challenge you face once your second baby has arrived and you are back home again, now looking after two children instead of one, is maintaining a steady routine of mealtimes and bedtimes. In fact, from the moment your second baby is born, you have to think about routines. Take feeding, for example. You have to decide whether to feed your new baby on demand (in other words, whenever she cries for food) or on schedule (in other words, at fixed time intervals even though she may appear to be hungry between these times). The same applies to sleeping, because you can let her wake and sleep whenever she wants, or you can encourage her to develop a sleep pattern so that she does the bulk of her sleeping during the night. And then there are your older child's needs to consider as well.

Juggling your day will be complicated. Your second baby's sleeping and eating times, for example, will not coincide with those of your firstborn's simply because the older child will sleep and eat less frequently. Nevertheless, after the first few months, you'll find that both children's natural body cycles will begin to coincide more and that's when you can begin to establish a similar regular routine for meals and bedtimes that suits both of them – this will certainly help you get through the day more easily.

Parents have different views about routines, especially when a baby is involved. You may feel that there is plenty of time to establish a routine when your baby is older and for now, she should be fed and attended to whenever she wants, or you may believe that your baby should follow a routine from the first moment because that makes life more predictable. Or, even if you were a flexible parent the first time round, you may find that with a second baby, adhering to a schedule will make your life easier. There's no intrinsic right or wrong answer – only what works for you! Most parents, however, do find that a routine is necessary for managing two children. There's simply so much to get through during the day when caring for a second baby and an older child that a structure of some sort is required.

A steady routine with both your children means you can plan your day with a bit of confidence. If

A TYPICAL DAY'S SCHEDULE

Every child is different and every family routine is different. Here's an example of a daily timeline for managing a four-month-old baby and a three-year-old child

6:30 am	baby wakes; older child is asleep
6:45 am	baby is changed and fed; older child is still sleeping
7:30 am	older child wakes and has breakfast; baby plays
8:00 am	baby plays while older child gets ready for preschool
8:45 am	older child is taken to playgroup, and baby goes along, too
9:15 am	baby is brought back home and plays
10:00 am	after feeding, baby has a nap
11:30 am	baby wakes, has a feed, then plays or goes on short outing
3:15 pm	older child is collected from preschool, and baby goes, too
4:00 pm	baby naps, older child plays and has snack
5:00 pm	older child has evening meal, and baby wakes up
5:30 pm	baby is fed while older child plays
6:00 pm	bath time for baby, older child plays
6:30 pm	bath time for older child, baby plays
7:00 pm	baby has last feed, and older child has milk
7:30 pm	both baby and child are tucked up in bed
8:00 pm	baby and toddler asleep – mother flops in chair!

you know, for instance, that your baby has a feed mid-morning and then again at lunch time, with luck you will have the time in between to do something else. In addition, you'll be able to get through the daily chores more easily because your older child and baby are likely to be more cooperative when following a routine. Their anticipation of the next event harnesses their enthusiasm and this helps you get through the day. The downside with a steady routine is that there is a possibility that your children become so tied to the routine that they get upset when there is a change. For example, your baby might howl the place down if she doesn't get her afternoon nap at the time she expects. You might then worry that you are driving a wedge between you and your baby by not giving her what she wants the precise moment that she wants it. You may be concerned that this will make her unhappy.

Psychological research suggests that children don't like extremes and this also applies to schedules. Having a routine that is totally rigid and unbending can be very restricting and can curb your children's liveliness but having no routine at all can leave them feeling insecure. It's a question of balance. Even if you have a routine, you don't have to be a slave to it. Things don't have to happen exactly on time every single day. Family life won't crumble if you are unable to manage the evening baths at the usual time nor will chaos ensue when you give your second baby an extra feed one day. A routine that is flexible increases your children's ability to adapt to change and enables you to respond to them more spontaneously. Bear in mind, also, that routines change with age – the schedule of mealtimes and bedtimes that you have for your little one at three months, for example, will have to be modified when she's six months anyway because of her rapid development.

Making a success of feeding

There is no doubt that breastfeeding wins hands-down compared to bottle feeding when it comes to health and nutrition. Research confirms that breastfeeding during the first year helps protect a growing baby from infections, allergies and other medical conditions. It's also true that many mothers don't breastfeed their new babies, either for practical, health or emotional reasons, and those babies thrive fully from successful bottle feeding. If you breastfed your first baby, you learned the practicalities and overcame difficulties so that establishing breastfeeding with your second baby shouldn't be too difficult. And, even if this new baby presents some challenges, your previous experience should stand you in good stead and you'll have some idea of who to go to for help. However, knowing the potential pitfalls of breastfeeding and the potential challenges that lie ahead, it may be that the prospect might not seem so appealing this time. If you have any doubts, remind yourself of the health benefits breastfeeding brings to your child. Think too, about how easy it is and how you don't have to worry about preparing and sterilising bottles. Remind yourself, too, that this form of feeding will only be temporary and before you know it, your new arrival will be drinking milk from a cup.

If you were unable to – or didn't want to – breastfeed your first child, but now want to do so for your second baby, don't let inexperience stop you! There are plenty of experienced professionals and parents who will be willing to give you advice. Speak to the nurses at the maternity hospital or at your local health centre. Read books on the subject or web-based articles about breastfeeding, and talk to other mums who you know breastfed their babies. It's never too late to learn, and you may be surprised how much less challenging it is than you imagined. Mothers who breastfeed are typically very willing to support those who are less confident with this method of feeding.

Don't let yourself be put off by others who may tell you that bottle-feeding is easier and that formula milk is better. People usually have very strong opinions about how best to feed a young baby, and if they fed their own baby by bottle, they may think they should persuade you to do the same, especially if you've done so before. Arguments from well-intentioned family members and friends about the advantages of formula milk can be very persuasive when you are tired, harassed and struggling. Don't suffer in silence. You'll feel better once you explain that you intend to breastfeed no matter what they say because of the health benefits for your baby and that they are inadvertently making you tense by their remarks.

Establishing breastfeeding

Whether or not you breastfed the first time around, this time, you have an additional complication – you have your firstborn with whom to contend. She may not be pleased to see her new sibling snuggled up so close to you, while she herself has to drink from a cup while sitting alone in a chair. She might need time to adjust to this, and in the meantime, you could find that whenever you start to breastfeed your second baby, the older one is always at your side, nuzzling in beside you, as if unconsciously trying to disrupt the process. Some first-born children choose that exact moment to "accidentally" fall and hurt themselves, forcing their mother to pay

them attention instead of feeding the baby; others can't help themselves from misbehaving, which is another way of expressing jealousy of the new baby's cosy relationship with their mother.

The best way to deal with this form of sibling jealousy is to prevent it happening in the first place. For a start, explain breastfeeding to your older child and point out that you fed her this way, too, when she was that age. Tell her about all the health benefits of breastfeeding. And don't exclude her at these times. There is no reason, for instance, why you can't sit and chat with her while you feed your baby – if you are relaxed about this, your older child will be relaxed, too. Alternatively, give her a toy or game to play with when you feed your second baby, so that she has lots to keep her busy. Let her "study" the breastfeeding process up close if she wants, so that there is no mystery. Using a breast pump to express milk means that your first child can bottle feed her young sibling occasionally, under your close supervision. If she understands breastfeeding, if she

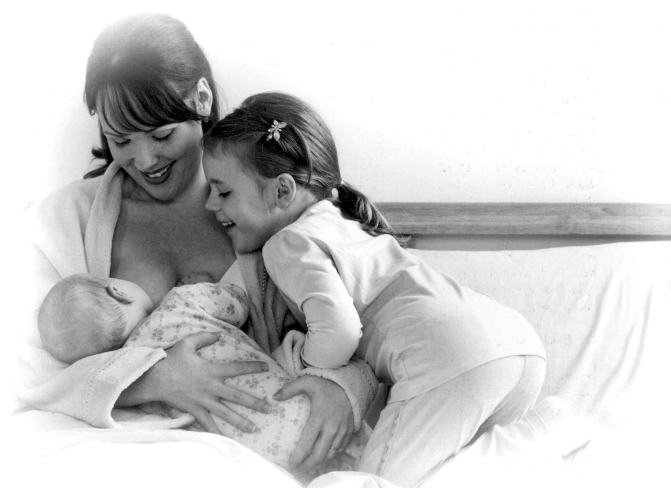

is connected to it in practical ways, and if she doesn't feel the need to be disruptive in order to compete for your attention, breastfeeding will be less stressful for everyone.

Think positively and have confidence in yourself and your baby. Even if you successfully breastfed your first baby, if you have any worries that this baby may not be getting enough nourishment or is failing to thrive, your family doctor or health visitor will be able to help. They or professionals they have recommended will be able to answer any questions you have about the practical mechanics of breastfeeding, about how best to position your baby and about how to stimulate the flow of milk. They will advise you on the rate of your baby's weight gain, and will alert you to any potential health difficulties that may be present. In the meantime, take an optimistic perspective, and work on the assumption that breastfeeding is satisfactory for her. Try to relax during feeding, as that helps the milk flow. Your baby senses your tension and as a reaction becomes tense herself, which in turn inhibits the feeding process. You'll quickly get to know your second baby's feeding preferences and adapt accordingly.

Make practical plans to share as much of the feeding as you can, within the limitations imposed by breastfeeding, otherwise you may start to feel tired and dispirited. Most parents find the first year of caring for their second baby very tiring, and breastfeeding adds an additional strain because mum has to be there all the time when her baby feeds. To reduce the pressure on you, you could ask your partner to feed your baby expressed milk, say in the evening so you get a good night's sleep, or that he look after your baby in-between feeds so that you can nap. Although your baby might resist taking milk from a bottle while being held by someone else, she will adapt eventually. It's good for her to get used to being handled by someone other than you; that helps develop her sociability and resistance, while giving you a much-welcomed respite from the normal feeding routine. And it will promote bonding between your partner and baby.

Out and about

After the first few days or weeks of family life with your second new baby at home and your older child full of energy and excitement, it's time to start thinking about having an outing with them, perhaps for a walk in the park, or a shopping trip to the local mall or a visit to one of your friends. It probably seems a good idea at first, but by the time you have everything prepared, got both children fully dressed and toileted in readiness for the voyage into the great outdoors, packed and loaded all the paraphernalia of child-care equipment for two and you are finally ready to leave the house, you may feel so exhausted that all you want to do is sit down and rest, never mind go out with your two children in tow! But don't give up at this point. Remind yourself that outings together are an important part of family life, providing excitement for your

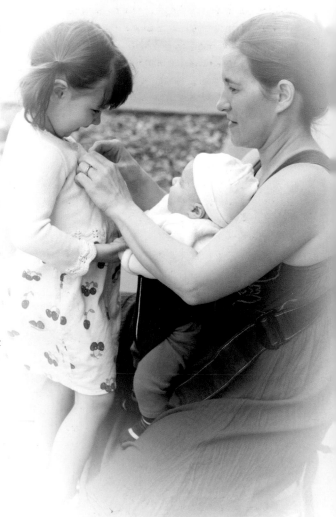

CHOICE OF OUTINGS

Typical outings for an infant under one year include the local park, a baby music or massage class, a mother-and-baby group, a shopping trip, meeting another mum and baby for coffee at home or in a cafe, and baby cinema (special morning feature movies for mums with young babies). And possible outings for an older child under the age of four or five include soft gymnastics or play, pull along toys in the park, a mother-and-toddler group, a dance class, arts and crafts activities, a swimming class, or story-telling sessions at your local library.

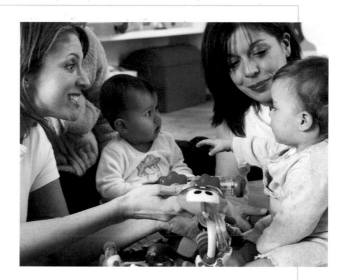

children, a focus for the next few hours and a chance for you to get to know each other in a different context outside the family home.

Advance planning is the key to a successful family trip. So check out your destination well ahead of your departure to make sure everything is as you expect. Have a clear idea about facilities for changing and feeding a young baby as well as what activities will be on offer for your older child.

It also helps to forget any notions you have of travelling light – that's for single people or couples without children. Work on the assumption that you should take everything you can carry. No matter how many clothes, pieces of equipment and spare nappies you take with you, the chances are that you'll find it is not enough. Err on the side of caution. Access to a car for an outing with your children means not only will you have door-to-door transport but also that you'll have lots of storage space. On a sunny day, you can bring wet-weather gear on the off chance that it might rain. You can also bring extra toys and any other babycare equipment you choose. You might end up using some or all of it, but if you don't use any of it, just pack it away again when you return.

The effort of preparing for the outing will probably be more than you imagined, especially the

first time you take both children out together, and you may get to the point where you think it is too demanding. Don't give up. Keep preparing and remind yourself that you and your children will have a great time; it will prove to be worth the effort. Allow yourself and your children plenty of time for all stages of the outing. Instead of leaving things until the last minute, start preparing, say, at least half an hour before you intend to step over the threshold. Likewise, assume that the journey time to and from your intended destination will take longer than usual because of all the loading and unloading of the children and their equipment.

Have realistic expectations for the outing. Don't be over-ambitious. Aim for short outings when your second baby is young – at least to start with. If you expect too much or attempt an outing that is overly ambitious, you'll end up disappointed and frustrated. A short trip of, say, no more than an hour may be just right for the first one. Keep in mind that the main reason for the trip – apart from having a break in your usual daily routine – is for you and your children to share each other's company and to have fun together. So do your best to stop the practicalities from becoming so great that the pleasurable part of the outing get pushed into second place.

Special parenting situations

Thinking about raising a single second baby can be sufficiently challenging but what if two come along at the same time? Now you have to raise three children, and two of them will have immediate needs. Or instead of your baby becoming part of the family right away, your second baby needs to stay in hospital, perhaps because she was born prematurely and needs supervision and support until she is stronger, or maybe because of a health problem that has emerged. Both of these situations will challenge you as a parent.

Twin considerations

The birth rate for twins has steadily increased over the past decade, mainly as a result of successful fertility treatment. (All ranges of multiple births have increased, not just twins, for the same reasons. If you imagine caring for, say, triplets or quadruplets, this will certainly help you to think that managing twin babies isn't that difficult after all!)

As you will discover, twins can be twice the usual expense and work but also twice the usual fun! And that makes family life very special for you, the twins and their older sibling. There are particular challenges for parents who have twins, simply because of the children's closeness in age, their special relationship, which is often more intense than normally found between siblings, and their underlying need to develop as distinct individuals despite being part of a twosome.

Twins are either identical or non-identical. When identical twins are conceived, a single egg, which is already fertilised by a sperm separates into two identical parts. Each part develops into a baby. Since each child comes from the one egg (monozygotic), these twins are always the same sex with the same inherited characteristics. When non-identical or fraternal twins are conceived, two entirely separate eggs are fertilised by two entirely separate sperm at the same time. Since each child comes from a different egg (dizygotic), these siblings are no more

alike than any brother or sister. Twins often occur as a result of fertility treatment because more than one egg has often been used in the process in order to increase the chance of a successful fertilisation.

Although identical twins look the same to most other people, there are always physical differences, however small, and you'll soon notice them. For instance, sometimes one twin is left-handed while the other is right-handed, which will lead to them developing different styles of handwriting. One twin may be smaller than the other or the twins may have significantly different personalities. Rates of development also vary. Twins, whether identical or not, can develop a secret language, one their parents may not understand. However, there are plenty of instances when two siblings – not twins, but close in age – also develop a similar type of secret spoken code. The birth of twins will have a great impact on your existing child, who may have been more stunned than you to learn there are two new babies in the family instead of one. As well as competing with two others for her share of your time, she may feel somewhat isolated and detached from her young siblings because they have each other – she doesn't have a sibling her age, but they do. It's important that your older child doesn't stand back and that she develops a strong relationship with each of them. Encourage her to play with each one of them alone and together, and maybe if she's old enough, to help care for each – say, amusing one baby while you change or feed the other.

Twins typically draw attention from other adults and children. There is something engaging about two sibling babies the exact same age, especially if they appear identical – a matching set is intrinsically more interesting and unusual than one on his or her own! You can be sure that your twin babies dressed the same for an outing to the shops or to the park will get a larger number of glances, stares and positive comments than your first born child ever did when you took her out on her own at that age. And while this extra attention is great for the recipients, spare a thought for their older sibling who may be totally dismayed that the twins get all the admiration and she is pushed into the sidelines. Self-esteem is vulnerable in these circumstances. That is why it helps to draw other people's attention to her as well whenever they try to focus entirely on the twins. The very fact that you bring her into the conversation is likely to lift her confidence and boost self-esteem.

Research has shown that twins often develop speech and language skills at a slower rate than non-twins, probably because they usually construct their own "shorthand" system for communicating with each other. That's why a broad range of language activities will be so indispensable for your twins. Most important of all, talk to them throughout the day as they progress through their routine activities. Read them stories, sing them songs and recite poems and nursery rhymes when you can. Encouraging their speech and language at this very early age gives them a head start. This could be something your older child could help with.

Even if you have identical twins who look alike in every way, each has her own individual characteristics, personality and interests. For instance, one twin might enjoy being cuddled by you when distressed while the other might prefer you to sing to her when she is upset. Try to meet these different interests and different temperaments, so that the individuality is allowed to develop. Another way to encourage your twin babies' individuality is by making an effort to spend some moments alone with each of them, rather than spending time only with them together. Easier said than done, of course. All it takes is a few minutes each day playing with one of your twin babies, while the other is either cared for by someone else or is asleep. Later on, each twin will have to learn to stand on her own two feet, and temporary separation from the other child has to happen at some stage. Often the start of playgroup, nursery or school is the point at which parents specifically decide to actively encourage their twins' individual identities.

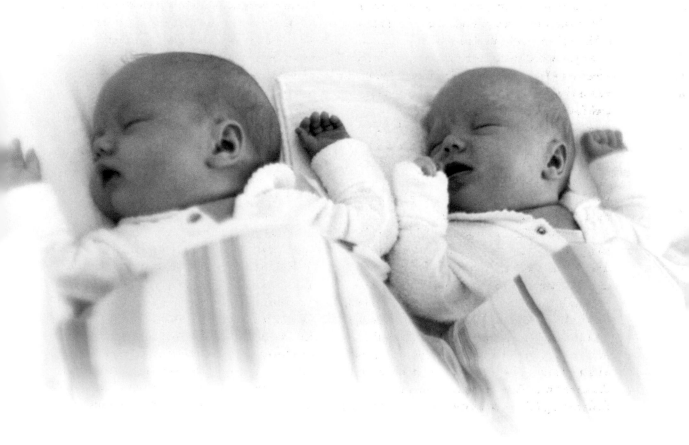

Few parents of twins, particularly identical twin babies, are unable to resist the temptation to dress them alike. They look too cute in their matching outfits, forcing any passerby to have a double take! That's fine, as long as it is not a symptom of a general parenting strategy that aims to strengthen their similarities at the expense of developing their individual differences. Identical dressing is harmless, fun and totally acceptable occasionally. If it becomes a matter of routine, however, you might want to think about your motives for doing so and to consider the wider impact this could have on your children's natural uniqueness as two distinct individuals.

Baby needs hospitalisation

Whatever the reason for your baby's extended post-delivery stay in hospital, you'll be anxious and stressed. It's not easy when one child is at home and the other is in hospital. Aside from all the health worries about your baby that you have to deal with, and the practicalities of running between both places, the hospitalisation and medical support is likely to interfere with the plans you had for your first born child to meet the new arrival.

Ask the doctors any questions that come into your mind about your baby's health. You'll only be able to relax and feel confident when you know, for instance, what's wrong with her, what treatment she requires, what the likely outcome will be, how long her recovery is likely to take and what treatment is involved. It might be a good idea to write all your questions down so that you don't forget anything when you are speaking to the professionals who are providing hospital care for your newborn baby.

Try to stay calm irrespective of the severity of your baby's health problem. If you are tense, your baby will sense this and become tense as well – as will your other child. In contrast, if you are calm and relaxed, your positive attitude will help promote your baby's recovery. This isn't a case of pretending that nothing is wrong, it's more about presenting a calm appearance on the outside even if you are extremely anxious on the inside.

Use lots of loving gentle touching with your baby in hospital whenever you get the chance. Gently stroking her cheek, holding her hand or smoothing her hair, helps soothe her and establishes the growing bond between you. Of course it would be great if you can pick her up and hold her close to you, and if you can breastfeed her, but that may not always be possible. Much depends on the medical problem and the type of treatment and support she receiving. Yet you can still have some skin-to-skin contact with a baby who lies on her back in an incubator with a feeding tube. Loving touch between you and her promotes her physical and emotional wellbeing in many different ways.

In the midst of all this stressful coming and going between home and hospital, your older child is trying to make sense of the situation. That's why the best strategy is for you to give her an honest explanation, one that is appropriate to her age and stage of development. Tell her that something is wrong with your new baby, but express this as positively as you can. For instance, if she is two or three years old, you could say "Your little sister isn't well. The doctors are giving her medicine to make her better". If she's four or five years old, you can provide more information, for instance, "Your little sister was born earlier than we expected. This means she needs to eat very carefully to make sure she grows properly. The best way for her to eat well right now is to stay in hospital".

Avoid any gory details about medical procedures and treatment, no matter how old your firstborn. Keep your explanation basic and accurate. Reassure her that her new sibling will soon be well and back home. In fact, the sooner she sees him in hospital, the better for everyone. Once your firstborn has a grasp of what's going on, and once she sees that the baby is a real person, she'll be more cooperative and understanding, which in turn will make life easier for you.

Involving your existing child

Family life will be so much more rewarding for your children and you when your children are strongly connected. A connection should start before your second baby is born and continue from the birth itself (see page 101). What happens in the early days and months can set the tone for your children's relationship with each other throughout their lives – that's why it helps when their tie is positive right from the start.

The most common age-gap between a firstborn child and her younger brother or sister is two years – and yet research has proved that an age-gap of two years between siblings is most likely to result in tension, jealousy and resentment. No wonder the typical two-year-old can be such a handful when the second baby arrives in the family. And when you think about it from your first-born child's point of view, her difficult behaviour is hardly surprising. After all, she's used to having you all to herself, and she wants that way of life to continue forever. She worries about having to share your time with someone else. She might also be afraid that you will love the new baby more than her, and that she will be less important to you, or even that you want a second child because she herself is not good enough for you or that you are having another baby just to punish her. In other words, she feels insecure.

Looked at this way, you can understand why she is unsettled by the news that a new baby is on the way, as well as the actual arrival itself. And she can show her anxiety in different ways. She might become clingy, tearful and moaning, or aggressive, hostile and uncooperative. It's the change in her behaviour that tells you something is wrong. As a parent, you know that loving your second baby won't decrease your love for your older child. But she doesn't know that. She has to learn by experience, which takes time. In the meantime, she may feel jealousy and hostility towards you and the new baby. So it's a good idea to involve your existing child right from the start (see page 116).

After delivery

When she visits your second baby in the hospital for the first time, try to arrange that you are not holding the new arrival. That way you can give your full attention to your first born. Give her a big cuddle, tell her how pleased you are to see her and ask lots of questions about what she has been doing since you last saw her. After a few minutes, introduce her to her younger sibling. Make sure the new arrival has a present lying beside him in the cot for his older sibling (one that you purchased previously and took into hospital with you) and arrange for your first child to take along a present for your second baby. This exchange of gifts is stage-managed, yet it can help form an emotional tie between the two children right from their first meeting, and reduces the likelihood of tensions between them later on.

One of the much-cited advantages of home births is that the first child is more connected with the delivery process. Her mum doesn't disappear to hospital while she stays at home with dad or gran, and she doesn't have to wait for news reports to find out what's going on! In that sense, a home birth can be good for establishing a strong relationship between a first and second child. Yet that assumes everything goes according to plan. A firstborn child who sees her mother in discomfort and pain, or who observes anxious professionals trying to problem-solve a difficult delivery, could possibly be resentful of the new baby who, as far she is concerned, is the cause of all the upheaval. There are no guarantees. Like all forms of childbirth, delivery at home needs to be carefully thought out from all angles.

When the baby's home

Once that initial meeting is over, get your older child involved in some of the minor chores of baby-care. She'll be full of self-importance when you ask her to bring you a clean nappy from the pile in the corner, or when you thank her for rubbing in some cream on the baby's legs after bath time. Basic tasks of responsibility make her feel part of your second baby's life.

The first few days when you are back home with your family after the birth of your second baby will normally be a very busy time, with visitors keen to see your new arrival. They can help your existing child keep any feelings of jealousy in check by bringing a present for her as well as one for the baby. Wherever possible, ask your visitors to do this and do try to encourage them to spend a few moments with your older child before they go charging in to see the baby. True, the main purpose of their visit is to inspect the new arrival, but there is no harm in quietly asking them to spend a

moment or two chatting to your other child first. And appoint your firstborn as tour-guide. She'll love to be given the job of leading visitors into the baby's room, and will take great pride in explaining all about him. This particular role ensures she gets lots of attention too, and emphasises that she is the "big one" at home – you'll find that she responds very positively to your request.

It's also important for you to maintain your relationship with your firstborn at the same time as encouraging her to have a strong relationship with her new sibling(s). One of the best ways to do this is by making sure you spend some time alone with your older child every day, perhaps while your partner is bathing your second baby or when the youngest is sleeping. A few minutes individual attention from you every day will make her feel that she is still as special to you as she was before her sibling came along. If your first child can continue her usual daily routine without the baby's schedule interrupting, for instance, going to playgroup or visiting her friend, then so much the better.

Your older child is very sensitive to your comments (and your younger one soon will be). Never compare your children to each other. When you lose your temper, you may inadvertently compare your older child with the new addition, perhaps pointing out that her younger brother never complains when his toys are tidied away or when it's time for bed. Such comparisons are always divisive, however, and will only make your firstborn resentful of you and of your second baby. Likewise, make allowances which recognise your first child is older, for example, by allowing her a later bedtime – a basic measure like that demonstrates to her that you recognise she is older and more mature, and this helps maintain your positive relationship with her.

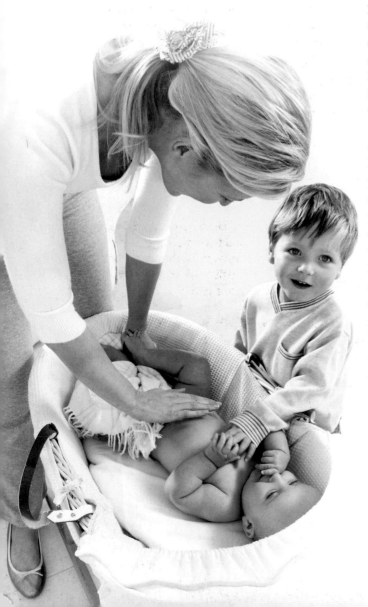

Looking ahead

Nothing stands still, not even parenting. There are fashions and trends in the way children are raised, and therefore attitudes and ideas about how to bring up children might have changed since your first child was a baby. For example, fierce debates continue to rage over whether parents should be schedule-based and be strict about their baby's sleeping and feeding patterns whether they should be more child-orientated and flexible. The range of babycare equipment and transportation devices might also have changed in the intervening years, as well as the types of toys now available for young babies. In every aspect of life, technology plays an increasing role.

Have an open mind and be prepared to listen, to read and to watch. You can still learn a lot about raising children from others. Even though you are an "old hand" at parenting, advice from other parents, grandparents, close friends, doctors and from anyone else whose opinion you might value can be very helpful, enabling you to make an informed choice about what to do. (And, of course, there may be people who give an opinion without being asked.)

There is a law of nature, which applies to members of your family who also have young children, and it is this: they are all experts in every aspect of raising a baby! In other words, they know all that there is to know about bringing up children (at least, that's what they think). The fact that their views are based on their own experience, and are influenced by their own personality and their children's personalities, doesn't stop them from expressing their advice to you about how to be a good parent in today's society.

No matter what the current trends are in parenting when your second baby arrives, and no

ways a second baby changes your life

While having a second baby means that there's one more person to love and who loves you, it's also true that you will

1 Be much more tired This is particularly true if your older child is an active toddler or if he regresses. Taking care of two children will take up most of your day.

2 Have less spare cash While you may be able to save money on some equipment and clothes, your second baby may end up costing you a lot more than your first. You may not be able to accommodate a new baby into your existing home as easily as you did the first and may have to stop working to care for both.

3 Have a lot more work to do In addition to taking care of and tidying up after two children, the differences in their ages can mean preparing different meals and arranging individual activities and outings.

4 Have less time in which to do things Feeding, bathing and dressing two children takes a lot of time as does taking them places and dealing with their differences. Moreover if one child becomes sick, you have the extra burden of care.

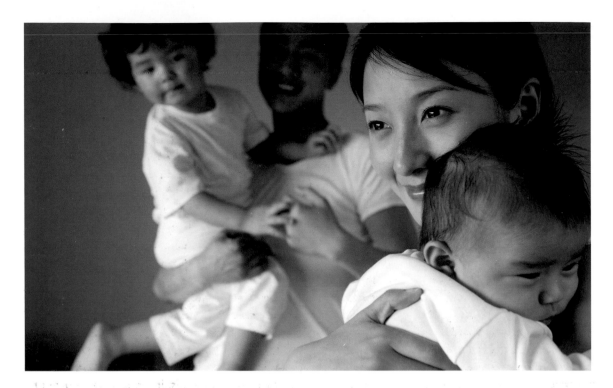

matter how much things have changed or remained the same since your first child was young, there is no 'right' way to raise your baby. True, there are universal rules about parenting, such as the need to help your baby fulfil her potential, the need to stimulate her through play, the need to love her and so on. However, there are plenty of ways to meet these needs, not just one. What suits one baby might not suit another. The fact that your sister's baby liked a musical toy does not mean that your baby will like the same toy. Every child is different, whether they are from the same family or not; what worked for your older child or your sister's children might have no effect at all on your second baby.

Living with two children

You have to make up your own mind about what sort of parent you want to be for your second baby. By all means, read about contemporary theories of raising a baby and talk to other parents who follow approaches other than those you are familiar with. But she's your second baby, no one else's, and the final choice of how you care for her rests with you. Anyway, you won't be able to implement advice that makes you

uncomfortable or that you won't be able to follow – for example, if a relative suggests putting your baby on to solids to help him settle at night, you won't do this if you think he's too young to digest solid food.

In the months and years that lie ahead, you'll have the delight of watching your first and second child grow up together. But that's not a passive process. How you manage them and contribute to their lives is the biggest single influence on the outcome of their development. Recognising and responding to their individual differences will be a key challenge for you – but if you achieve this, it will be highly rewarding for you and for them.

Your first and second child will vary in temperament, personality, likes and dislikes and possibly gender. One might have an easy and relaxed manner and deal calmly with everything that comes her way, while the other might be tense and volatile, quickly upset by the trivial challenges in life. One might be very outgoing with a particular interest in drama and dance, while the other may keep to her room, listening to music and reading. One might excel at her studies while the other excels at athletic endeavours. You'll be surprised at times at how two children from the same family, with the same home environment and the same upbringing, can appear so entirely different from each other! And even when they appear to like the same things, their different abilities and personalities may produce widely differing results. That's the nature of child and family development.

Aspire to fairness not equality

Do your best to respond to your children as individuals. Aim for fairness in your parenting rather than equality. Equality occurs when both children get the same, whether or not they want it. For example, you might decide that since you bought your first child a piano because she asked for piano lessons, your second child should also have piano lessons at the appropriate age. After all, you already have the piano, so it would be cost effective for your second child to repeat the pattern. That would be equality. In this instance, however, fairness might mean your purchasing a drum kit as your second child chooses this musical instrument to learn to play, despite the fact that her older sibling learned to

play the piano. Or maybe you would offer ballet or drama lessons if your second child is not interested in learning an instrument.

Fairness isn't always possible, as often there are practical and financial considerations to take into account, yet it is worth aspiring to. Perceived lack of fairness is a common complaint of siblings – the cry of "She always gets more than me" is heard in most families at one time or another – and is one the main causes of sibling jealousy although there are other factors, too. In fact, sibling rivalry is so common in virtually every family that most psychologists now regard it as normal. You can rest assured that your children are not the only ones to fight with each other – you would have great difficulty finding two young siblings who never fought with one another.

Yet the intensity of sibling jealousy varies from family to family, and even within the same family; some children are more antagonistic towards a particular sibling. Usually, it simply comes down to the individual differences between the first- and second-born, whether in personality, talents and

GENDER DIFFERENCES

Boys (compared to girls) tend to...
- Enjoy risk-taking and be adventure-seeking
- Take part in rough-and-tumble play
- Use their hands as a first response to conflict
- Take longer to develop language and independence skills
- Compete with one another when playing together
- Have a better developed right side of the brain (hence advanced spatial skills)

Girls (compared to boys) tend to...
- Weigh up risks carefully before taking action
- Like sedate activities, such as puzzles and creative play
- Resolve disagreements through talking
- Start talking and achieve bladder control earlier
- Cooperate with each other during play
- Have a better developed left side of the brain (hence advanced speech)

abilities, gender, or even birth order. No matter how hard you try not to compare them with each other, the chances are that they will compare themselves spontaneously or that other people will compare them (for instance, friends and relatives) and if one child is cleverer or more talented than the other, then their relationship may suffer. Each child must feel valued and that she does not have to compare her achievements against those of her sibling.

When making major decisions as a parent, you instinctively act in the best interests of your children. Yet that doesn't mean your children will like your suggestions, for instance, when you don't let your three-year-old play with another child because you think that child could have a negative influence on her. And neither do you probably like being a parent who has to say "No" to your child. Have confidence in your decisions, even in the face of opposition from your child or when having to balance long-term considerations against a disagreement with your child in the short-term. That responsibility goes with the parenting territory.

You may find that you want to change some aspects of parenting with your second child, having learned from experience with your first. For example, you may be less exacting about rules for bedtime because you now know that an extra five or ten minutes won't cause any significant upset. Whereas you were a stickler for time keeping with your first child, you have a more relaxed time-keeping approach with your second. There's nothing wrong with that. You don't have to feel guilty because the way you respond as a parent has changed through time. You don't have to feel bad because you wish you had done things differently with your first child. You did what you thought was best at the time. If it turns out that in hindsight you can now see alternative courses of action for managing your second child's development and behaviour, that's a positive sign of your personal growth – it would be much worse if you didn't learn from experience.

BIRTH ORDER DIFFERENCES

First born tends to seeks adult approval and does her best to please; however, she may have difficulty expressing her feelings and tends to be easily upset.

Second born is often interested in the new and unconventional, preferring creative activities rather than science; she often has a sarcastic sense of humour.

Middle born tends to be the one most likely to seek a compromise in a dispute – she tends to be the diplomat in the family.

Youngest child often has a lower regard for rules, frequently challenging her parents and others who try to establish discipline.

Only child can have difficulties when it comes to sharing, cooperating and turn-tasking with her peers, but this usually improves quickly with experience

Dealing with sibling rivalry

Sometimes you'll feel that you cannot win, no matter how hard you try. There will always be moments when your children become locked in a dispute because of their jealousy towards each other. Although you cannot eliminate sibling rivalry altogether, you can try to control it.

Treat your children seriously. If they think that you regard them with amusement rather than genuine respect, then they will soon become even more jealous of each other. Listen to their complaints, even though the endless list of gripes and groans about their siblings can be extremely irritating. It is better to make time to listen to what they have to say – if you do try to ignore them, they will force you to give them attention by fighting with each other. When you have heard their complaint, suggest a solution. For instance, if they

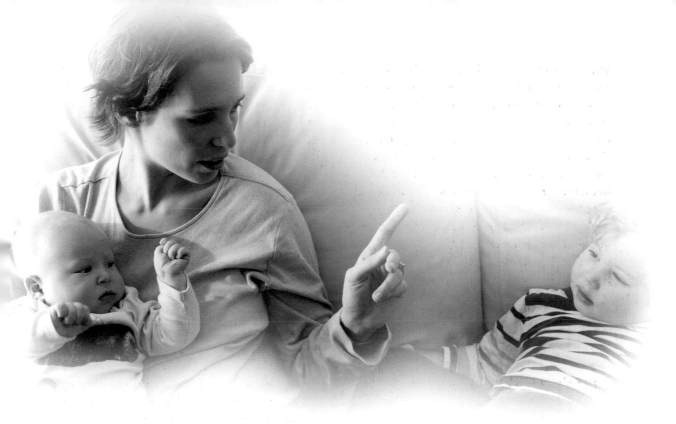

both want to play with the ball, organise them so that one plays with it for five minutes and then it is the turn of your other child.

Later on when they are older, you might find that their arguments centre around the fact that the older child is allowed more freedom than the younger child – this is especially common when the younger one is around the age of five years. Like it or not, he has to face the fact that his sister is older and is therefore entitled to do some things that he cannot, such as going to bed later than him or being given more individual responsibility at home. Point out the significance of their age difference.

The positive relationship between your children can be enhanced by teaching them how to cooperate more with one another. For example, you can provide opportunities for sharing. Many sibling fights start because one or more of the children is unable to share his or her toys. Your children will learn how to do this with practice, however, so don't make all the decisions about sharing for them – ask one of them to share out a bag of sweets, and see how she gets on. Show your children how to cooperate, if necessary. Give them a small household

chore that requires them to work together in order to complete the task (such as putting the cutlery on the table). If they begin to fight with each other over who should do what, explain that one child can put out the knives, another the forks, and so on.

Partner considerations

Having a second baby also has an impact on your relationship with your partner. True, you already have experience of the massive change that took place when your first baby arrived – you shifted from being a couple without children, able to make lifestyle and work choices that suited you and your needs, to a couple with children, now having to make child-centred decisions. So you know what it is like to put a baby's needs before the needs of you and your partner, and presumably have adjusted accordingly.

With your second baby, there will be further change – perhaps not as dramatic as with your first baby but change all the same. There will be less space in the house, there will be less money to go round, your career and work plans will be on hold once again, and the practical demands of caring for two children are simply greater than when caring for one. All of these have an impact on the relationship with your partner. Family stresses can strengthen the connection between parents but can also create barriers between you. Successful parenting is heavily influenced by, amongst other things, the type of relationship you have together, your expectations, resilience and capacity to adapt to change.

A settled family life does not depend on the practical arrangements you make, for instance, whether it's you or your partner who gives your children their bath tonight, or whose turn it is to make dinner. Neither is it a question of your financial arrangements, for instance, whether you have enough money to afford to pay for a baby sitter and a meal out, or what you need to sacrifice in order to pay the utility bill. Nor is it reliant on your agreeing about your extended family, for instance, whether you should go to his parents with the children this weekend or to yours, or which relative you should invite to your older child's forthcoming

4 ways to improve shared child care

Some new mothers find it difficult to share babycare. They may feel they are better at caring for the baby and that only the best is good enough. If you are so inclined, be aware that discouraging your partner from helping with feeding, changing, dressing and bathing your baby, may cause your health and relationship to suffer. You may become so fatigued physically and emotionally that it won't be good for you or your baby. Bear in mind that if you think your partner's child care skills are not up to scratch, practise will only make it better!

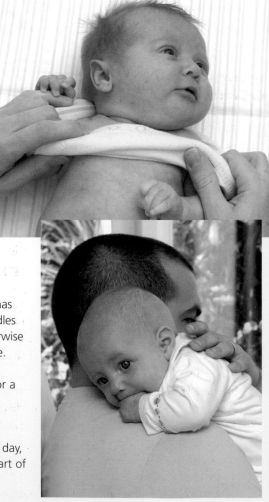

1 **Be specific about what you need** Instead of generalising about how tired or overworked you are, agree with your partner specific tasks you each will perform. Of course, it's best to ask him to be responsible for those things he prefers to do or is good at instead of assigning chores.

2 **Try not to criticise** what your partner is doing. Everyone has his/her way of approaching things and if your partner handles your baby or child differently than you, just accept it, otherwise you'll give him reason not to do the task at all in the future.

3 **Remember to thank your partner** and to offer praise for a job well done.

4 **Relate the day's news** It's important to tell your partner about what your new baby and older child did during the day, especially if he works away from home, so that he feels part of family life when he's not around.

birthday party. All these factors play a part in your home life, but the central component when it comes to partner consideration is honest and open communication between the two of you.

If you are able to express your ideas and feelings openly to each other as parents, adults, and partners, then resentments are unlikely to build, misunderstandings are unlikely to occur and your relationship is more likely to remain positive and optimistic. Making time to talk with each other is crucial. Try to avoid the trap of becoming so absorbed in the demands of parenting that you and your partner lose sight of each other as a couple. When communication with your partner becomes low on your list of priorities, the chances are that problems will emerge. In contrast, good channels of communication mean that most potential problems can be resolved before they reach crisis point.

When you don't agree

Perhaps the most worrying type of disagreement about parenting is when you and your partner are in dispute about the best way to handle your children. As you have already discovered, managing children is not an exact science! Everybody has his or her own opinions about topics such as discipline, bedtime routines, how to deal with tantrums and so on, which is hardly surprising given that there is usually more than one way to do anything. But problems can arise when serious differences of opinion occur between parents over how to raise their child (although do bear in mind that minor disagreements about child-related issues are perfectly normal).

Sustained disagreements between you and your partner about bringing up your first child and new baby can create inconsistent parenting. At every age, your children need a consistent structure at home, a predictable set of rules, which they are expected to follow. If you tell them one thing and your partner tells them another, there no consistency whatsoever. This confuses them, and could start to make them feel anxious. In addition, serious parenting disputes affect the atmosphere at home. You feel tense, your partner feels tense, and before you know, your children feel tense, too. In a strained environment

like this, tempers become frayed. Soon everyone in the home will have a higher level of irritability and bickering.

Not only that, children can be manipulative. A young child can be quick to exploit differences of opinion. When she doesn't get what she wants from you, she will immediately rush over to your partner in the expectation that he will be more obliging. Your toddler is only interested in achieving her goal, and she'll approach the parent most likely to give in to her. You can't blame her for using a loophole that you and your partner created for her and her sibling. For all these reasons, you and your partner should resolve your disagreements about the way your children should be raised, as quickly as possible.

Resolving differences

First, make a sensible and responsible agreement that you won't fight about your children in front of them. Aside from the fact that they definitely don't want to hear the two of you fighting with each other, your children need family rules and routines to be clearly set out. Witnessing the two of you having argument about, say, whether or not your second baby should be allowed to have an extra feed during the afternoon, simply makes your older child feel miserable.

Second, listen to what each other has to say, even though you may dislike what you hear. Parents form their views on child care in a number of ways. For example, you might want to be lenient with your children because that was the way you were brought up and you have happy memories of childhood. Or maybe you want to be lenient because you had a very strict upbringing, which you didn't like and therefore you want things to be different for your own child. Or perhaps you think a lenient approach is better because you think that your children are more likely to love you than if you are more authoritarian with them. Your partner's views also stem from a variety of sources. So attend to each other's views about parenting principles.

Make time together, just for the purpose of talking about these matters. Once you have both had your turn to say what you think, spend time

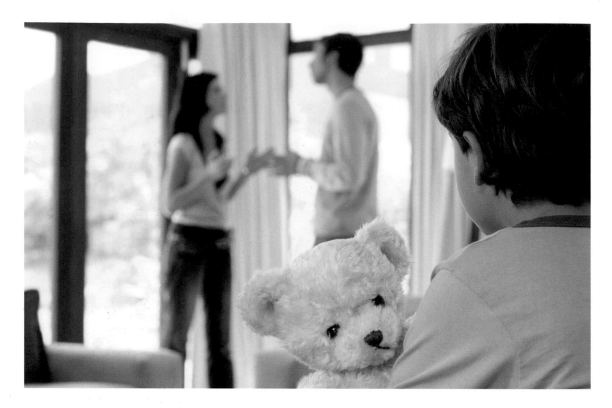

discussing the source of your differing opinions. Consider your own childhood and the ways you were brought up by your parents. This will help you understand why you are fighting about how you manage your children, and will form the first step in resolving the differences – and it will bring you closer together, instead of driving you apart.

Having agreed to settle your differences when your children aren't within earshot and having tried to understand why you and your partner fight over them, the next step is to resolve the conflict sensibly without unnecessary confrontation. Together, you should consider the strengths and weakness of the various alternatives. Be honest; don't reject your partner's ideas just because you didn't think of them first. Accept that your way is not the only way.

Suppose, for instance, that you and your partner fight over your second baby because you think it's time she should be encouraged to hold her spoon when eating while your partner thinks she should continue to be fed by an adult. Talk through the pros and cons of each approach. You'll probably find that there is merit in both strategies. Eventually,

however, reach an agreement on what to do. This might be that for one week she holds the spoon for the first mouthful of each meal, then gets the rest of the meal fed to her; the second week, she holds the spoon herself for two mouthfuls, and so on, gradually extending the amount of food she takes independently. Carry this out for a period of, say, three weeks. Make a commitment that during this time that you'll both support the approach, and that at the end of the three-week period you will evaluate its success. If the strategy has worked, then you can justifiably be pleased with yourselves. If it hasn't been effective, then make a further commitment to try another approach for a couple of weeks.

This process of negotiated trial-and-error is far more helpful than you and you partner constantly fighting over the way your children should be raised. Two parents working together create will a far more satisfying relationship for them and their children than when they are in opposition.

Index

Acknowledgements

Illustrations
Amanda Williams

Suppliers
Thanks to the following companies for supplying products/photography:
Clearblue for the Ovulation Prediction Kit, p15.
Fertility Scope for the Saliva Fertility Test, p15.
theBabaSling™ for the carrier, p60.
Mothercare, for equipment shown, p69.

Photographs
Professor Stuart Campbell p35, p38, p39 and p40.

Photolibrary.com
p19, p27, p28, p46, p47, p50, p53, p55, p56, p57, p63, p67, p68, p70, p72, p81, p84, p99, p100, p103, p104, p106, p110, p113, p116, p118, p121, p124.

Science Photo Library
p44 Health Protection Agency, p79 (left) Dr H.C.Robinson, p79 (right) Mike Miller.

Getty Images
Jacket

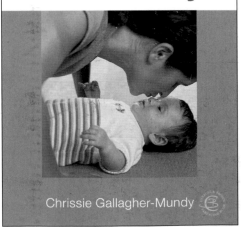